CRACKING THE CROSSFIT® OPEN

*How to Outperform Your Peers
in Every Workout*

OLIVER NORRIS

Cracking the CrossFit Open
How to Outperform Your Peers in Every Workout

Copyright © Oliver Norris, 2018
All rights reserved.

Editor: Christina Roth
Cover Design: Sarah Smith

ISBN: 978-1-5218-8511-6

Published by STC Press

Contents

Introduction

My aim with this book is to help you improve faster in the sport of CrossFit. After reading it, you will have the tools you need to develop more strength, power, and skill in every movement. This will enable you to perform better in all workouts—particularly in the CrossFit Open. But before we get into the details, I want to tell you how this book came about, and how you can best use its contents to your advantage.

Why I wrote this book

How can I improve myself in CrossFit? How can I outperform my peers? And how can I place higher in the Open? Soon after I started CrossFit, questions like these drove me to search for increased knowledge. I read countless books, blogs, and journal articles about health, training, sport, and fitness. My aim was simple: to improve faster.

This search was disappointing and frustrating at first. The vast amount of knowledge available on these subjects is scattered, confusing, and often conflicting. There are entire books and websites devoted to completely opposite views. Some authors attribute these contradictions to a difference in "philosophies" or "schools of thought." To me, such attributions reflect a lack of commitment to get to the bottom of things. Fitness is a physiological state, so actual facts should exist about which training methods are most effective.

After digging deeper, I started to see patterns emerge in the chaos. Some underlying principles of CrossFit are derived from older sports with more established training methods. Other principles come from scientific studies published only in recent years. And yet others are based on the experience of some of the world's leading coaches. In these three areas, I finally found valuable and established truths. Ever since, I have used these insights to progress more rapidly than my peers.

This book contains those truths. It is the guide I wish had existed when I started on this journey. It organizes what I have found in a holistic way for athletes who want to improve faster. The book will enable you to do so, without first going through the same time-consuming search as I did.

No matter where you stand, this book will help you progress in the sport of CrossFit. If you are a beginner, most of this will be new to you. If you have more experience, some concepts will be familiar, but the way they connect and support each other will be novel.

But why should you listen to me? I am not an elite athlete. Before CrossFit, I had never practiced a sport for more than a few years. I had been in and out of various gyms, never lasting more than a few months. I got into CrossFit at 27 and have practiced it for only two years, so I am by no means an authoritative figure when it comes to the sport. But I believe that this is actually a benefit to you for a few reasons.

First of all, my search and commitment to the sport have resulted in a high rate of improvement. Since starting CrossFit, I have participated twice in the Open. The first time I placed around 130,000 on the Leaderboard and the second time around 50,000. This was out of approximately 200,000 male competitors and one million male athletes who train regularly. So, I went from a limited sports background to the top 5 percent of CrossFit athletes in a short amount of time. This is the goal of the book: helping you improve fast—no matter where you begin.

Additionally, advice from someone in a similar position is often more useful than advice from those with much greater experience. This fact is well known in the domain of mentors and mentees. Consider an entrepreneur in the first stages of a startup. That person will benefit the most from advice given by those who recently faced similar challenges. Advice from the CEO of a large company, who faces different challenges, will be of limited use.

In CrossFit, we can see examples of this principle. Professional athletes often emphasize pushing themselves as hard as possible. This is more applicable to athletes already performing at the highest level of the sport. For the majority of athletes, though, other factors are more important—for example, building consistency, optimizing training load, and balancing the different aspects of training. These factors help intermediate athletes improve faster than going all-out in workouts every day.

Third, I have kept this book free of any goals other than to help you improve. I am not affiliated with any products, and there are no links to a website where I ask you to buy my training program or additional materials. And Oliver Norris is a pen name, not my real name, because I do not wish to use this book to make a name for myself or build a platform to sell other products. The advice should speak for itself, regardless of who wrote it.

Unfortunately, this is seldom the case with the best CrossFit athletes and coaches. You only need to view their Instagram profiles to see that much of their advice is actually meant to provide them with income, not help you improve. ("This supplement/gadget has helped me so much to improve! Use the coupon MYNAME30 to get a big discount when you buy it.") Instead of following such recommendations in the hope of reaching the fitness level of these individuals, you are better off reading unbiased advice.

Finally, you don't need to take my word for it. This book is based on scientific knowledge and the experience of experts—both from CrossFit and other sports. This means my task is more so that of a journalist than a coach. My aim is to gather the most helpful insights on how to improve your performance in one place.

What you should know before reading

In this book, I assume that you have a basic knowledge of CrossFit and its key terms. But in case some concepts are unfamiliar to you, I have included a Glossary of Terms at the end. Start by reading through it. If you are unsure about the meaning of a specific term, you can look it up there for clarification.

For any guide like this to be effective, a good framework is paramount. The framework should include all factors that are both significant and relevant:

Significance: There is an endless number of factors that affect our athletic performance. Athletes looking to improve should focus only on the factors that are significant. This can be hard for many due to the lack of organized information in the world of athletics.

For example, commercial interests constantly promote supplements that have limited or no beneficial effect. The same applies for clothing, equipment, and gadgets. This bias, combined with a lack of knowledge about how training works, leads to many athletes losing track of the fundamentals. This book focuses only on factors that significantly affect your athletic performance.

Relevance: We define these significant factors as either controllable or uncontrollable. Controllable factors include your training methods, your mentality, and the foods you eat. Uncontrollable factors include your genetic predisposition to athletics, training experience, and biological age.

Too many athletes worry about uncontrollable factors, complaining about their age or genetics. This is a waste of both time and energy. Such thoughts will only disempower you and make you defeatist in your attitudes. This guide focuses on how you can become the best version of yourself. Uncontrollable factors are irrelevant on that journey.

By focusing only on factors that fulfill both of these criteria, this book will allow you to ignore irrelevant information and therefore clear up your thinking. It also makes you focus on things you can control. Both will make the task of improving easier.

The book is divided into three parts:

1. **Approach:** This part shows you how to approach the sport mentally. This includes your strategy and tactics when it comes to performing, plus your motivation and attitudes.

2. **Training:** This part explains how to train for the fastest improvements. It covers the underlying principles, how to ensure sustainability, and the most effective training methods to develop skills, strength, and conditioning.

3. **Recovery:** This part explores how to enhance your recovery and improve between training sessions. It provides recommendations for nutrition, lifestyle, and supplements.

After reading this book, you will have a holistic view of the things that matter most for improvement. After that, it will be up to you to act.

PART I: APPROACH

Thought precedes both action and results. The outcome of everything you do depends on how you approach it mentally. The first part of this book will equip you with the mindset needed to be effective in your training. It will give you the three things you need to succeed on the path of improvement. First, the path should lead in the right direction. Second, it should be a good route to follow. And third, you should have the motivation to walk the path.

Chapter 1: Strategy

Most sports have predetermined rules and objectives. In basketball, athletes play for 48 minutes with the aim of scoring more points than the other team. Training for the sport means improving the things that help the athlete achieve this aim. This could include technical drills, conditioning, strength development, and practice matches.

CrossFit differs from such sports in two ways. First, before competing, athletes cannot prepare according to predetermined rules and objectives. In the CrossFit Games, workouts are generally announced when athletes should perform them. This means there is little or no time to prepare for a specific challenge.

Second, CrossFit is not only a sport but also a philosophy for improving general fitness. Accordingly, workouts are designed to reflect the principles of this philosophy. Athletes looking to do well in the sport of CrossFit should know the philosophy as well. This enables them to be better prepared for the workouts they will encounter in the future.

These two differences make the sport of CrossFit unique. I would also argue that they are key reasons for its fast growth. In most other sports, the health benefits are only a side effect. Improved health is not the goal but rather winning according to predetermined rules. The health benefits from CrossFit, on the other hand, are the goal itself: the fittest person, in the broadest sense of the term, will do best in the sport.

My aim with this book is to help you improve your general fitness, which is tested in both workouts and competition. But this aim is still too vague. What exactly constitutes general fitness? And how should we train to achieve it?

This is where the CrossFit Games come in. This competition is where the sport and the philosophy of CrossFit come together. Held every year, the Games are open for anyone who wants to take part. In 2018, 500,000 athletes participated—an increase of 120,000 from the previous year. The Games are designed according to the CrossFit philosophy by testing fitness in the broadest sense of the term.

For the vast majority of participants in the CrossFit Games, the aim is to perform as well as possible in the first stage: the Open. The Open is where athletes of all levels test their abilities against thousands of others around the world. From the Open stage, only a handful of athletes proceed to the Regionals, the next stage of the Games. Accordingly, this book focuses only on the Open stage of the CrossFit Games.

We begin the journey by analyzing past Open workouts. I have analyzed every Open workout from the last five years to gain insight into what matters most to do well in the competition. Later on, these insights will guide you in choosing the best training methods to prepare.

Focus on specific time durations

First, one of the stated goals of CrossFit is to improve fitness across broad time domains. This is a very general prescription for training. It could mean anything from a 10-second sprint to a 17-hour Ironman triathlon. We need a more specific definition. The best way to get that is to view the time durations of Open workouts in previous years.

The following chart shows the duration of each Open workout in the last five years.[1] Each bar represents a past workout, and its height shows how long it took to finish it.

---

[1] In the CrossFit Open, one workout is published online every week for five weeks in a row. Athletes have three days to finish and submit a score for each workout.

Workout Duration

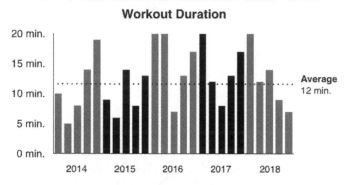

Note: Some past Open workouts had a time cap, which is not a good indicator of the actual duration, as most athletes finished in a shorter time. In those cases, the median athlete finish time is used as a more representative time duration. Specifically, this is done for workouts 18.5 (median finish time of 7 min.), 17.5 (17 min.), 17.3 (8 min.), 16.5 (17 min.), 16.2 (8 min.), 15.5 (13 min.), 15.2 (6 min.), 14.5 (19 min.), 14.2 (5 min.), and 13.5 (4 min.).

As you can see from the chart, almost all workouts for the previous five years have been between 7 and 20 minutes long. This means that the stated broad time domains span only 13 minutes in practice. Each year contains a mix of workouts of all durations, with an average duration of 12 minutes.

The best training plan will prepare you for peak performance within these time durations. You will need the power to work at high intensity in the shorter workouts. And you will need enough endurance to sustain high performance for up to 20 minutes.

Increase your power

Another way to analyze past workouts is by their goal. The following chart shows a count of past Open workouts, organized by the goal athletes were ranked on.

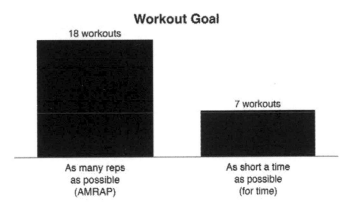

Interestingly, the goal of every Open workout is to either perform as much work as possible within a specified time frame or finish the required work as quickly as possible. These are actually two sides of the same coin. According to this, every past Open workout has essentially shared the same goal: do the work as fast as you can.

Categorizing the workouts by the type of goal shows us that the Open is a test of how much power we can generate within 7- to 20-minute time frames. In this book, we define power as the time-rate of work. In other words, power is the amount of work performed within a specified amount of time.[2]

Combine different movements

Another characteristic of past Open workouts that we can inspect is their structure, or how the workout is organized into different movements. There are four primary types of workout structures in past Open workouts:

- **Couplets.** These are workouts with many rounds and the same two movements in each round. An example of a couplet would be 5 rounds of 10 burpees and 40 double-unders.

- **Triplets** are like couplets but with three movements in each round.

---

2 Power can unfortunately mean different things in the context of fitness, depending on which source you read. Definitions of terms should always be clear to avoid confusion. In this book, I use the same definition of power as is used in physics. When you read about power in later chapters, it will always mean the time-rate of work.

- **Ladders.** These workouts feature a weightlifting movement in which the weight becomes heavier with each round. An example of a ladder workout would be as many rounds as possible of 5 squat cleans, adding 20 lb. on the barbell between each round.

- **Chippers.** These workouts do not have any rounds. Instead, athletes perform movements in succession. An example of a chipper workout would be 100 pull-ups, 200 push-ups, and 300 squats, performed for time.

The following chart shows past Open workouts categorized by these four structures. One insight we can gain from this is similar to that of the goal categorization: power is the main predictor of performance. Additionally, the four ladder workouts indicate that strength can be the dividing factor every now and then.

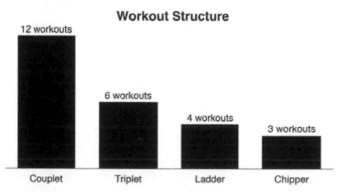

Note: Past ladder workouts also include some elements of couplets and triplets, making them a test of power as well as strength.

Another interesting insight from this data is the prevalence of couplets and triplets. This shows how CrossFit combines different movements to increase intensity beyond the stress of any single movement. We will take note of this and mimic it to some extent in our training, discussed later in the book.

Improve the right movements

We cannot simplify CrossFit down to only maximizing power and combining a few movements. This becomes clear when we look at the frequency of movements in past Open workouts. The following chart shows the frequency of each movement appearing in an Open workout for the last five years.

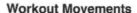

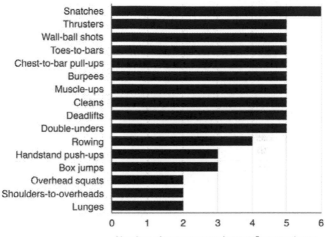

Note: Different variations of similar movements are grouped together for simplicity. This includes the power and squat variations of snatches and cleans, ring muscle-ups and bar muscle-ups, and dumbbell and barbell variations of lunges, cleans, and snatches.

We can see that past Open workouts consist of 16 different movements. Being able to perform every single one of these movements should be your priority. Focusing on power is of little use if you cannot meet the requirements of the workout. Furthermore, if you want to do well, you should also learn to be efficient in executing these movements.

The Open has shown us how a weakness in any one of these movements undermines performance. In 2018 for example, the third Open workout (workout 18.3) included both bar muscle-ups and ring muscle-ups. The year before, workout 17.2 included bar muscle-ups.

And the year before that, workout 16.3 relied heavily on bar muscle-ups. Not having the ability to do muscle-ups would have sidelined you in a workout every year for the past three years.

Another insight from this breakdown is that the variety of movements in the Open stage is smaller than many people may have thought. Compared with the Regionals or the Games, the movements are few. For example, in 2018, every single workout movement had appeared before. The only exceptions were the handstand walk, which appeared so late in workout 18.4 that most athletes didn't reach that point.

This narrower pool of movements is presumably for the simple reason of practicalities: movements need to be simple to equip and simple to judge. It would be difficult for all 13,000 CrossFit boxes to accommodate many of the movements. Similarly, movements with ambiguous judging standards would cause problems for those who need to assess whether each repetition should count.

It follows that training for the Open can be focused movement-wise. While legless rope climbs, pegboard mounts, sprints, and sled pushes can be fun, our main focus will be on the movements listed in the chart.

Finally, some movements are more frequent than others. The most popular movement, with six occurrences in the last five years, is the snatch. Immediately following are nine more movements, all with five occurrences. These are thrusters, wall-ball shots, toes-to-bars, chest-to-bars, burpees, muscle-ups, cleans, deadlifts, and double-unders.

Rowing comes after these Top 10 movements, with four occurrences. Handstand push-ups and box jumps follow, with three occurrences each. Finally, overhead squats, shoulders-to-overheads, and lunges trail with two occurrences each.

This indicates the relative importance placed on these movements in the Open. We can use this insight to choose which movements to focus on. Accordingly, we should schedule the most frequent movements more often in our training.

Train for the right modalities

We can also look at past workouts in terms of broader categories of movements, so-called *modalities*. This gives us an overview of what type of training we should be doing. CrossFit consists of four key modalities: weightlifting, gymnastics, conditioning, and calisthenics (also called body weight movements).

The following chart shows the number of past occurrences of every movement, categorized into these four different modalities.

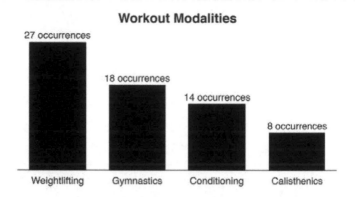

Workout Modalities

27 occurrences

18 occurrences

14 occurrences

8 occurrences

| Weightlifting | Gymnastics | Conditioning | Calisthenics |

Note: Each Open workout contains multiple movements. Hence, the total occurrence of past movements is higher than 25 (the total number of Open workouts in the past five years).

From this we can immediately see that the Open revolves in large part around weightlifting-related movements. Not far behind are the various gymnastics movements, and last, conditioning- and calisthenics-related movements are also important.

This reflects the cross-training element that is included in the word "CrossFit." We should make sure that our training is varied in terms of different types of movements. This way, we will be ready to tackle the varied workouts when the Open season begins.

Develop your strength

Finally, past Open workouts indicate the weights we need to lift, giving us a better idea of how much strength we should develop to perform well in the future. There is no single metric for strength, as the movements and rep schemes can be very different. Instead, I have highlighted all strength-heavy movements from the last five years. Reading through this list should give you some indication of the strength you need to do well:

- **18.4:** Varied couplet with 21-, 15- and 9-rep sets of deadlifts at 315/205 lb. (143/93 kg)

- **18.2a:** 1-rep-max clean

- **17.4 and 16.4:** Chipper starting with 55 reps of deadlifts at 225/155 lb. (102/70 kg)[3]

- **17.3:** Couplet/ladder ending with three squat snatch singles at 265/185 lb. (120/84 kg)

- **17.2:** Modified triplet with dumbbell lunges and power cleans at 50/30 lb. in each hand (22.5/15 kg)

- **16.2:** Triplet/ladder ending with 7 squat cleans at 315/205 lb. (143/93 kg)

- **15.4:** Couplet with ascending reps of cleans at 185/125 lb. (84/57 kg)

- **15.1:** 1-rep-max clean & jerk immediately following a triplet

- **14.3:** Deadlift ladder ending with 35 reps at 365/225 lb. (166/102 kg)

So, 10 out of 25—or 40% of all workouts—have included heavy weights. Without adequate strength, you are likely to be stopped dead in your tracks in at least one

---

3 The two numbers indicate the prescribed weight for men and women, with male weight appearing first and female, second.

or two workouts each year. It follows that strength development should be a part of Open training for many athletes.

Summary

In summary, here are the key insights derived from analyzing past Open workouts:

- **Time:** Duration of 7–20 minutes, with a 12-minute average.

- **Goal:** The workouts test power—i.e., the amount of work performed over time.

- **Structure:** Workouts combine multiple movements, mostly two or three for repeated rounds.

- **Movements:** Sixteen different movements have been tested—all more than once.

- **Modalities:** Of the four modalities, weightlifting is the most common. Gymnastics, conditioning, and calisthenics are prominent as well.

- **Weight:** 40% of workouts require significant strength.

Having gone through this analysis, we now know better what to train for. A training program for optimal Open performance should maximize three parameters:

- **Conditioning:** Maximum power output in the 7- to 20-minute time frame
- **Skills:** Efficient execution of the 16 key movements
- **Strength:** Adequate strength to move heavy weights

We now understand the tests we may encounter in future Opens. In other words, we understand the playing field. But no less importantly: how do the players we compete against behave? And what are the best tactics to outperform our peers? This is the focus of the next chapter.

Chapter 2: Tactics

A defining characteristic of CrossFit is its emphasis on measurability. One expression of this is the Open Leaderboard. The Leaderboard publicizes the score of every athlete in every workout. This data gives us valuable insights when analyzed with the aim of maximizing your Open success. Three insights stand out in particular: finish the workouts, work on your weaknesses, and raise your standards.

Finish the workouts

Submitting a score for five workouts may sound easy. But when push comes to shove, your resolve will be tested. In my experience, Open season comes with two waves of mental resistance: the first during the registration period, and the second halfway through the workouts.

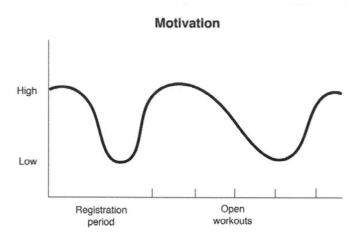

The first wave is registration resistance. When it comes to actually registering, a part of you will not want to sign up. Your mind will conjure up all sorts of justifications. You have been feeling sick for the last few weeks. You are in much worse shape than before. You have a minor injury. You made travel plans during the Open season. You cannot find a judge. It is too much with everything else going on in your life right now. You will be in much better shape next year.

All these perceived reasons are actually justifications your mind is making up to resist change. Participating in the Open pushes your limits for five consecutive weeks. The pressure in Open workouts is higher than for the regular WODs, so the Open workouts will cause you more discomfort than you are used to. With the prospect of being pushed outside of your comfort zone, your mind will resist.

Your first task when it comes to the Open is to see this resistance for what it is. Becoming better in the sport is going to be uncomfortable. Having this awareness will make it easier for you to recognize the resistance when you encounter it so you can ignore it and move forward.

Additionally, there is another challenge you need to overcome. When forming new habits, whether with CrossFit or anything else, most people experience a "honeymoon period" at first. During this time, you'll have the strongest resolve and enjoy performing the new routines. After that, there comes a second stage, when the new habit ceases to be fun and instead feels like a burden. The most difficult part of habit formation is to get through this second stage.

In the Open, this stage is the second wave of mental resistance. You may be excited to perform the first one or two workouts. But in the later weeks, your motivation may decrease. The workouts will seem like a chore, and a part of you will wish you could go back to your regular routine.

Just like with registering, you can get through this low-motivation stage by ignoring the resistance and doing every workout anyway. If you do that, your excitement will build up again as you reap the rewards of sticking to your plan. Then, when it comes to the final workout, you will be both happy and proud of yourself for overcoming both obstacles.

"Eighty percent of success is showing up." This quote by Woody Allen is remarkably accurate for the CrossFit Open. Approximately three million athletes currently show up for WODs on a regular basis. Of those, 500,000 signed up for the 2018 Open. This means that by registering, you have guaranteed yourself a place in the top 20 percent of all athletes.

To be sure, some do WODs only for the long-term health benefits and are not concerned with the Open. But in my experience, many who do not register regret it once the competition has started and their peers are competing.

These individuals then resolve that they will participate next year. But when the next year rolls around, they are still unable to overcome the mental resistance. The only difference now is that the "reason" isn't the same as last year's.

In addition to registering, posting a score for all five workouts will get you further still. As you can see in the following chart, approximately half of those who registered for the 2018 Open submitted a score for all five workouts. Simply by finishing what you started, you will already be above average in the competition.

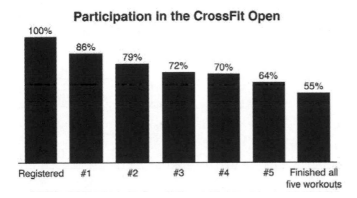

Participation in the CrossFit Open

Registered — 100%
#1 — 86%
#2 — 79%
#3 — 72%
#4 — 70%
#5 — 64%
Finished all five workouts — 55%

Note: This data is for the 2016 CrossFit Open. The numbers are similar for other years as well.

The fact that you are reading this book demonstrates that doing well in the next Open is something you care about. When the time comes, be aware of these two waves of mental resistance and resolve to overcome both of them. Never let your mind convince you to abandon goals that are important to you.

Work on your weaknesses

In 2015, CrossFit HQ introduced a new feature in the Open. That year, every workout came in two versions: RX (or "as prescribed") and Scaled. The Scaled version made the Open accessible to more athletes by reducing the weights and replacing complex movements with simpler ones.

This feature immediately proved popular. In 2015, the majority of athletes performed the Scaled version of at least one workout. As a consequence, Scaled workouts were included again in 2016, 2017, and 2018. The Scaled workouts remain popular and will most likely continue in future years.

This popularity means that performing the RX version of all five Open workouts will help your ranking. This is because Leaderboard scoring is set up in such a way: a single rep of the RX version of a workout counts more than any number of reps for the Scaled version of that workout.

Accordingly, aim to perform the RX version of all five workouts. To be able to do that, you need to have two abilities when the next Open begins: the necessary skills for every movement, and enough strength to move RX weights. This will ensure that you can stick to the RX versions of the Open workouts and finish above those who scale their workouts.

For many, this is easier said than done. Two common weaknesses in CrossFit keep too many athletes away from the RX version of Open workouts: lack of skills, and lack of strength.

Weakness #1: Lack of skills

The most difficult movements for most athletes are CrossFit's challenging gymnastics movements. They demand a high degree of both strength and skill at the same time. These include muscle-ups, bar muscle-ups, handstand push-ups, and toes-to-bars. Mastering these will set you apart from many of your peers when the next Open season arrives.

One of the best examples of such a divider is the muscle-up. In 2016, workout 16.3 was a 7-minute AMRAP consisting of 10 light power snatches and 3 bar muscle-ups. Sixteen percent of the men couldn't perform a single bar muscle-up. They posted a score of 10 reps, finishing only the first set of snatches and spending the rest of the time unsuccessfully attempting a muscle-up.

For the women, the number was even higher: 57 percent posted a score of 10 reps. Clearly, getting a single bar muscle-up would have put an athlete over tens of thousands of their peers in that workout.

Note that this principle of big Leaderboard benefits from mastering a difficult movement does not extend to all gymnastics movements. For example, you do not need to learn the butterfly technique instead of the kipping technique to do well in the Open. Although it can save you some time and grip strength, it will not get you over any workout bottleneck like the muscle-up will.

Addressing your weaknesses when it comes to the key gymnastics movements is more important. Focus your skill training on the handful of movements that have been demonstrated to affect Leaderboard placement significantly. We will discuss these movements in the training chapter later in this book.

Weakness #2: Lack of strength

Some Open workouts test weightlifting strength. Most years have featured some version of a ladder workout, with increasing weights in each round. This type of workout separates athletes based on their ability to move heavy weights. Including the ladder workouts, a third of workouts require significant strength. This means athletes who are strong will reap benefits in the Open.

One example of this was seen in Workout 16.2, a squat clean ladder combined with toes-to-bars and double-unders. For the women, the weights were not a limiting factor, but for the men, they were. The biggest separator was a set of 13 squat cleans at 185 lb. (84 kg). Seven percent of the men stopped where the set started. Another 33 percent stopped before finishing the set. A strong athlete can finish a set like this quickly, but 40 percent of the male athletes were stopped by either taking too long or not finishing a single rep.

This illustrates that strength is a weakness for many athletes in the Open workouts. A good training program should build adequate strength to move heavy weights as required in the workouts.

The benefits of workouts as prescribed

To see how helpful learning all the movements and building the necessary strength will be, we can look at Scaled vs. RX statistics. For the men, 19 percent scaled at least one workout in 2018. For the women, 52 percent did. After you've decided to register and perform all the workouts, your next task is to separate yourself from this group in the Open.

By mastering the Open movements and building up your strength, you will move even further up on the Leaderboard. In the next chapter, we will examine the most effective method for doing this. But before we do that, there is one final lesson to learn from athletes' past performances: the advantage of raising your standards.

Raise your standards

Athletes tend to obsess over workout announcements during each Open season. Which movements will be included? How long will the workout be? Will it include barbell work? Many ask themselves questions like this, eagerly awaiting the next announcement.

When the athlete then performs the workout, the focus is on achieving some mental goal appropriate for that person's fitness level. This could be finishing a set number of rounds or finishing the workout under the time cap, for example.

This is a flawed approach. Success in the Open, like many other competitions, is determined by relative performance. In other words, the only thing that matters is your performance compared to other athletes in your division. So, instead of obsessing about the playing field, those wanting to do well in the Open should focus on outperforming their peers.

A clear example of this was seen in 2017. Workout 17.1 tested mental toughness just as much as it did fitness level. The workout was a couplet consisting of alternating dumbbell snatches and burpee box jump-overs with a time cap of 20 minutes. This combination causes intense discomfort that needs to be endured for a long period.

As a consequence, most athletes focused on finishing barely under the time cap, usually by less than a minute. The aim for many seems to have been to be able to say they finished the workout, while minimizing discomfort by barely meeting the requirement.

This illustrates an important point. The fact that so many finished just under the time cap meant that the gain from barely finishing, as opposed to having a couple of reps left, was limited. However, the difference between coming in just under 20 minutes and just under 19 minutes was large. With most focusing on the 20-minute time cap, finishing in just 1 minute less was one of the biggest opportunities available for a jump on the Leaderboard.

So the final insight is: set your standard a bit higher than you usually would. If you think you can manage 3 rounds, aim for 3 rounds and 3 more reps. And if you think you can barely finish under the time cap, aim to be one minute below. The psychological factor in most Open workouts is significant, so defining a goal like this beforehand can help you separate yourself from your peers.

Chapter 3: Psychology

If you are not a professional athlete, there is a significant risk that none of the advice in this book will help you. Most amateur athletes eventually suffer from decreased motivation, and many drop out completely as a consequence. So before going into the training methods themselves, I want to provide you with strategies to prevent this and ensure you keep training for a long time.

I started CrossFit by attending a mandatory beginners' introductory course in my box. The class contained 30 people—old and young, fit and unfit, and everything in between. Our coach started the first class by saying that 80–90 percent of us would not complete the course and show up for WODs upon completion.

I was sure that he was exaggerating. After all, the course was only four weeks long. Why would most of us, all determined to improve our fitness, waste money on this course by not even finishing it and putting it to use? This seemed very unlikely.

But it turns out that the coach was right. Two months later, only two others and I had completed the course and attended a WOD with the regular members. The other 27 were nowhere to be seen.

Later, I asked one of the owners of our box about the high drop-off rate. She said that the drop-off rate was not particularly high at all. Whether I compared this to other sports or other CrossFit boxes, 90 percent drop-off rates or more within a few months is the norm for beginners.

To combat this, the box provides a deep discount for those who complete the course and sign up for a membership. They also survey the dropouts to see whether the course was too difficult, whether it was not to their liking, or if the box could improve the sign-up process.

It turns out that most of those surveyed liked everything, but they stopped attending because they didn't have enough time—usually due to family or work demands. The fact that you are reading this book means you have already overcome this cutoff point. But it still shows the tremendous force of inertia you are facing.

It takes energy to do everything, and so ceasing an athletic activity means you save your energy in the short-term. Conversely, in the long-term, the opposite is true: those who are fit have higher energy levels than those who aren't fit. But when you are building the habit of exercise and starting to move, you will face major resistance.

I managed to overcome this resistance, going from a limited sports background to consistent training four to six times per week. What follows are the strategies I have learned to sustain a high level of motivation. I divide these strategies in two parts. The first are practical strategies: adjusting your environment so you stay motivated. The second are mental strategies: thinking in a way that keeps you on track.

Practical strategies

- **Have a gym buddy.** Commit beforehand to going to the box with somebody at a certain time. If you lose motivation to train, your commitment to that person will keep you from skipping the session. This was the most important strategy for me. I cannot count the number of workouts where my commitment to my workout partner kept me from staying at home.

- **Log every workout.** By logging each time you attend, you start building momentum, which motivates you to keep going. Since I started, I have regularly updated a chart of my attendance each week. Looking at the chart motivates me to keep the momentum going.

- **Find the best time.** When I had time-consuming work commitments, I started going to morning classes at 6:30 a.m. This way, nothing could get in the way of attendance. When things came up later in the day, like prolonged meetings at work or family responsibilities, I was already done with my workout. During more relaxed times, I have gone at noon or in the afternoon.

- **Identify with the community.** For the first few months, I didn't see myself as a "CrossFitter," just an outsider doing the workouts. But I consciously started immersing myself more in the community. This included going to social events at my box and attending local competitions as a fan. This helped me lose my cynicism and reservations about the sport and embrace it more fully. As a consequence, it became more fun to attend WODs because I also looked forward to getting to know the other members better.

Mental strategies:

- **Trust your future self.** Let's say you wake up and don't feel motivated to go after work. Take the gym bag with you anyway, just in case. Often, you will find that as the day passes, you start to actually want to go and will end up doing so.

- **Just show up.** When my motivation was the lowest and I wanted to skip a workout, I set the goal of simply showing up at my box. After I showed up, going to the class was not an issue anymore since I was already there.

- **Think about afterward.** For the first year, there were many times when I didn't feel like training. However, there hasn't been a single time when I regretted training after the workout was over. Visualize the future by imagining how you'll feel after the class has finished: will you regret that you didn't go or be happy that you went?

- **Take responsibility.** If everything fails and you do not plan to go on a given day, don't rationalize or demonize your decision. Don't justify it by telling yourself you don't have the time or energy. At the same time, don't criticize yourself for not going. Instead, take responsibility and live up to the fact that you have decided not to go that day. This increases your sense of control, empowering you to decide differently next time.

In the last few years, psychology has provided great insight into the formation of habits. One of the most popular books on the subject is The Power of Habit by Charles Duhigg. In his book, he describes the dynamics and principles behind our habits in a constructive manner.

One particularly helpful term Duhigg has coined is the notion of keystone habits. These habits have positive effects on other areas of your life. Training is an example of a keystone habit. It increases your energy for other activities, makes you choose healthier foods, and helps you sleep and feel better.

I have found CrossFit to be very much a keystone habit. Realizing the positive effect of WODs on other areas of my life has kept me motivated to keep showing up for workouts despite not "feeling like it" on some days.

Gradually, after showing up consistently for over a year, an interesting change occurred regarding my motivation: it became difficult for me not to train regularly. Now, if I cannot go for a few days, I feel an urge to show up again, to get my blood flowing, to raise my fitness levels, and to eat, feel, and sleep better again.

Thus, mental resistance gradually disappears as the status quo becomes training instead of staying at home. But because this process takes months, or even years, the risk of dropping out before that happens is large. Hopefully the strategies I have outlined will help you get all the way there

PART II: TRAINING

Training is the catalyst for physiological improvement. Accordingly, how you train will receive the greatest attention in this book. In this part, we will first review the most relevant principles of training from science and expert coaches. Then, we will cover the things you need to do to stay consistent, most importantly by preventing injury. Finally, armed with this knowledge, we will determine the optimal way of training for rapid improvement.

Chapter 4: Principles

After reading the previous chapters, you are likely motivated to get started. In a perfect world, you would take your newly armed insights, look online for the perfect training program to excel in the next Open, and implement what you find.

Unfortunately, when it comes to improving physical performance, this will not work. There is an overload of information on the best methods to achieve this, much of which is conflicting. Furthermore, the insights available are so scattered that it is impractical for most athletes to put them to use.

For example, one day somebody in your box might tell you that the fastest improvements result from six or seven WODs per week. The next day you might read online that three or four workouts per week is an optimal frequency for recovery. A week later you might read that you should be "strength-biasing" your programming. But when you ask around about it, someone may say that this is an ineffective approach.

On top of this, you have companies trying to convince you that you need to buy various products to improve your results. You see advertisements for apparel, equipment, and mobility tools. On top of that, you have the supplements—protein, creatine, BCAA, and pre-workout and recovery drinks are all supposed to help. You see others at your box using these products. Not knowing how much they matter for improving—or whether they matter at all—you also buy them and hope for the best.

This combination of disorganized information and commercial interests results in skewed information on the principles of training. As a result, many athletes end up focusing on superficial things while giving the fundamentals less thought.

Unearthing the principles of training

Not long after I started CrossFit, I became frustrated by this misinformation. Much of the advice the people in my box were following seemed anecdotal and contrary to the knowledge I was gaining myself. I was unsure of what to believe.

This drove me to educate myself. Over the following months, I read various articles, including scientific journal articles, and textbooks on sports science and biology. Additionally, I read everything I could find from the world's best coaches in related sports. My goal was to find out which principles were the most important and effective in improving performance. Just as important, I wanted to identify the advice that didn't matter or that could even hurt performance.

During this journey, I found myself sharing these insights with other people at my box. Over time, these conversations became more frequent as I answered more and more questions, both from myself and from others. I became a training journalist of sorts, spending much of my time doing research and sharing what I found out. Finally, I decided to organize everything I had learned in one place for anyone to use by writing this book.

One of my most important goals for this book is to keep it completely free of any bias. I do not subscribe to any historical "school of thought" in the world of sports science. As previously mentioned, my sports background before CrossFit was unexceptional, with a few years of soccer, martial arts, and globo gyms under my belt. Additionally, I have not partnered with any company to promote any product. As a result, the information here should be as unbiased as it can be.

With that background, let's dive into the advice you need to boost your performance. To start, we will review the most relevant concepts on which we'll organize our thoughts about training.

Five principles of training

We can learn much about training for CrossFit using established principles from sports science. The last two decades of research have been especially fruitful, providing athletes and coaches with many insights widely used in sports training today.

However, locating this information in plain English and making sure not to confuse it with older myths still circulating can be challenging. The purpose of this chapter is to remedy this.

There are five concepts in particular that are both established and important for you to know as an athlete. These are adaptation, overtraining and detraining, training load, adaptation types, and periodization. These core concepts will lay a foundation of knowledge that we will build upon in later chapters.

Adaptation

Humans adapt to their environment. As a part of this adaptation, your fitness level continually adjusts to your level of physical activity, the quality and quantity of your foods, and various other environmental factors.

You change your fitness level by changing these factors. Your body then adapts by changing your physiology accordingly. This adaptation is continuous, which means the process never stops.

In sports science, the training adaptation model illustrates how this process works in the context of our fitness level. The model consists of three stages. The first stage is *training*, where you stress and fatigue your body. The second stage is *recovery*, where the body repairs the tissues affected and adapts by raising your fitness level. The third and final stage is *detraining*, where your fitness level gradually declines back to where it was before training.

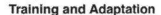

Training and Adaptation

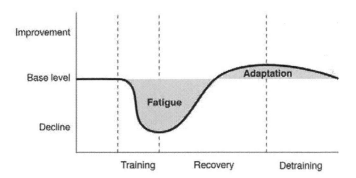

As seen in the chart, there are two effects at work during this three-stage process: fatigue and adaptation. Your fitness level first declines as you train. This effect is called fatigue. Then, your fitness level rises to respond to the training. This effect is called adaptation. Both effects last for a limited amount of time. Your fatigue fades away as your body recovers, and your adaptation fades away until you train again.

The conclusion from this model is that for peak performance, we should train at the highest point of adaptation from our previous training session. Training consistently at this "sweet spot" would result in a gradual increase of your fitness level, as seen in the following chart.

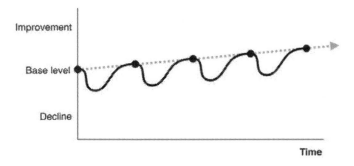

Over- and detraining

From the adaptation model, we can see that any deviations from the optimal training frequency will slow improvement. Train too early, and you will fatigue yourself again before the higher fitness level has been reached. Train too late, and your fitness level has already declined back toward the baseline. We call the first situation *overtraining* and the second *detraining*.

For optimal results, we need to be careful to do neither of the two.

This is not as simple as it seems. Physiological adaptations to training vary in duration. Replenishing our muscles' energy storage might take only 10–12 hours, but reaching the highest adaptation level might take one to three days. Muscle damage from strength training demands longer recovery than fatigue from aerobic training. Neurological adaptations when learning new movements will be of yet another duration. And adaptation of ligaments and bones takes yet a different length of time.

Furthermore, the time needed for recovery changes depending on our age and training experience. Older or more inexperienced athletes will need longer recovery times. Those who are younger or more experienced can train more often. Finally, optimal recovery duration depends on both the *intensity* and *volume* of training. Intense or long training sessions demand longer rest periods than more moderate ones.

In summary, the human body is so complex that no formula can determine an optimal recovery duration between training sessions. You will need to find your unique recovery time by experimenting on your own.

Always keep in mind the principle of "use it or lose it." Never wait longer than necessary between training sessions or you will impede your improvements. At the same time, overtraining also has a negative effect. It will deplete your physical and mental energy and require prolonged rest periods.

One of your key tasks is to find the optimal amount and frequency of stress to put on your body. The extent of this stress is commonly referred to as training load.

Training load

You will always need to be the judge of your training load, or how intensely you should be training. But to do so, it helps to have a useful framework to think about how much stress you are subjecting your body to. One of the best ways to quantify this is with the Training Load Factor (TLF) framework. It decomposes training load into three components:

- **Frequency:** The number of training sessions within a period
- **Volume:** The amount of training time during each training session
- **Intensity:** The intensity of each training session

In the framework, the product of multiplying these three components together is the Training Load Factor. Mathematically, the equation is as follows:

Training Load Factor = Frequency x Volume x Intensity

A good way to think about this equation is that you can choose two components to emphasize and one to sacrifice. If you want to train six or seven days per week, or even twice per day, you need to reduce either the volume or the intensity of each session. But if you stick to a lower frequency of three or four times per week, you can make each session count more by working long and hard each time.

All athletes use a combination of these three components to reach their desired training load. Even at the elite level, you will see this trade-off. Some athletes take few rest days, one or less per week, but keep the training volume lower on each day. Others take at least two strict rest days per week but train long and hard on the other days. Another common trade-off is within the day. Some athletes train in two or three shorter sessions, while others stick to a single longer session.

Additionally, you can lower intensity to accommodate a higher volume and frequency of training. Many athletes do this by using some sessions to practice skills at low intensities. Another method of lowering intensity is through active recovery days. On such days, an athlete might jog, swim, or row at an easy pace. These types of training sessions are much less taxing on the body and can even aid recovery.

No matter how you break down the three training load components, do not apply the same training load as more experienced athletes. Training age is a powerful determinant of the amount of load your body can handle without overtraining. As your experience increases, you will build up tolerance to a greater amount of load. This is especially important in CrossFit, where much of your training will be at high intensity. Such workouts stress both your muscles and your nervous system more than you are probably used to. Gradually increasing your training load over time is important for long-term results.

When it comes to managing your training load, your task will be twofold. First, you must find the appropriate Training Load Factor for the fastest long-term improvement. Second, you must determine the best mix of frequency, volume, and intensity to achieve this factor. You need to find out both by experimenting.

Start by estimating this factor on a weekly basis to visualize your current training load. Then change the components and see how you feel. To give you an example, let's say you attend four workouts this week, each consisting of a 20-minute session with an average score of 7 on a subjective 1–10 intensity scale. This would give you a Training Load Factor of 35:

Training Load Factor (35) = Frequency (4 sessions) x Volume (1.25 hours) x Intensity (score of 7)

If you feel like you could have done more that week, try raising the factor to 40–45. You do this by increasing the frequency, volume, or intensity of your workouts the following week. At some point, you will feel like the training load is too much to completely recover from, both mentally and physically. Then you can decrease it again to a more sustainable level.

Three dimensions of adaptation

As we previously discussed, the body adapts to the stress it is subjected to. But adaptation differs by the type of stress involved. There are three *dimensions of adaptation* when it comes to fitness: energy systems, intensity, and physiology. Understanding how to use these dimensions will help you train more effectively.

Dimension 1: Energy systems

The first dimension is energy systems. The body uses three different systems to metabolize energy and generate power: the phosphocreatine, glycogen, and oxidative systems. Each system serves a different purpose. The first system, phosphocreatine, generates explosive power for a few seconds. The second, glycogen, generates high power for slightly longer, or up to two minutes. Finally, the third, oxidative, provides lower-power energy for long periods, up to many hours.

We will not dive further into how these systems work, as the details are not necessary to know unless you are curious. What you need to know is this: effective training for general fitness will stress all three systems to make them more efficient. Ignore one or two, and you will be at a disadvantage for certain types of activities.

One of CrossFit's advantages as a fitness regimen is how well it trains all three energy systems. This is achieved through Metcons, or metabolic conditioning sessions, which are a critical component of most WODs. Metcons are workouts where a task is completed as fast as possible. For example, every Open workout for the past five years has been a Metcon.

Metcons are designed to train these energy systems, often all three simultaneously. Anyone who has tried a challenging couplet or triplet knows this feeling. Everything is taxed at once. Your strength depletes (phosphocreatine), your muscles tire (glycogen), and you are completely out of breath (oxidative) at the same time.

Effective CrossFit training taxes all three energy systems on a regular basis. This makes the systems adapt to higher stress loads over time. The level of adaptation of your energy systems is commonly referred to as your conditioning. If you deviate from regular WODs at your box, make sure to keep developing your conditioning with well-designed Metcons on your own. We will discuss ways to do this in chapter 6.

Dimension 2: Intensity

The second dimension of adaptation is intensity. In competition, we perform at the highest possible intensity to get the best results we can, be it speed, power, or strength. But when preparing for competition, we should not necessarily *train* in that zone. Training only at the highest intensity will quickly lead to injury or burnout.

For conditioning, we usually vary intensity already with our WODs. On some days, Metcons are tough, and on others they are more manageable. When you encounter the easier ones, you probably don't feel like you are achieving much. However, you actually improve other aspects of your conditioning when training at lower intensities. This is better for your long-term results than performing every Metcon to the point of nausea.

The same principle applies to weightlifting. When we lift weights, different adaptations take place in both the muscles and the nervous system. Many of these adaptations occur at lower intensities, at weights below 80–90 percent of your 1 rep max.[1] For the greatest

---

1 For further reading on this topic, along with more detailed information about neuromuscular adaptations to strength training, I recommend the book Periodization Training for Sports by Tudor Bompa.

strength gains, train using a wide range of intensities. Only a part of your lifting should be at the highest loads.

This is contrary to what many beginners do with the barbell. They often limit their weightlifting to maximum weights in the 1–5 rep range, which also limits volume and leaves out a part of the potential adaptations. In contrast, most experienced athletes mix higher- and lower-intensity weightlifting work, allowing for greater training volume and strength gains in the long term.

If you are too focused on maxing out every time you lift weights, change up your routine and make sure to also train using higher-rep schemes. This will develop your muscular endurance, or your ability to translate your strength into higher-repetition situations. Muscular endurance is important for performance, both in the Open and in regular WODs.

Dimension 3: Physiology

The third and final dimension of adaptation is physiology. Our body adapts to training in different ways physiologically. Weightlifting favors so-called structural adaptations. After heavy barbell movements, the body adapts structurally to the heavier loads, such as by repairing and growing muscle tissue. This process demands longer recovery between sessions.

On the other end of this dimension, skill development depends primarily on neural adaptation. During this process, the nervous system improves coordination, balance, and skill. Neural adaptation requires less rest between sessions than does structural adaptation.

This means that we can train skills more frequently than doing weightlifting. We will incorporate this principle when we discuss programming later on.

In summary, we should make sure that our training covers the whole spectrum of these three dimensions. Conditioning should stimulate all three energy systems regularly. Weightlifting loads should vary. And skill training should be more frequent than weightlifting sessions. Incorporate these principles and see your results improve faster than before.

Periodization

Periodization is a formal way to describe how you schedule your training. In its simplest form, periodization consists of cycles repeated over time. The most popular type of periodization in CrossFit is the "three on, one off" schedule. In that arrangement, the training period spans four days. The first three contain one training session each, and the fourth is a rest day.

In the three on, one off schedule, four days make one *microcycle*. This is the smallest cycle your training program contains. More commonly, microcycles are one week in duration. A weekly microcycle makes training consistent with our other life commitments. A common weekly microcycle in CrossFit is as follows: three training days in a row, followed by one rest day, followed by two more training days, followed by another rest day.

A Common Microcycle

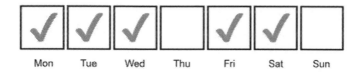

Mon   Tue   Wed   Thu   Fri   Sat   Sun

In most sports, elite athletes group these microcycles into *mesocycles*. Each mesocycle is usually between 4 and 10 weeks in duration. Specific milestones are set for the end of the mesocycle.

These mesocycles are then combined into one *macrocycle*. One macrocycle usually lasts for one full calendar year. The macrocycle is scheduled around a certain event, usually a competition.

In CrossFit, most elite athletes use these three cycles to structure their training. Often, the first few months following the Open consist of mesocycles with a greater emphasis on strength and skill development. When the Open draws closer, the emphasis shifts more to conditioning.

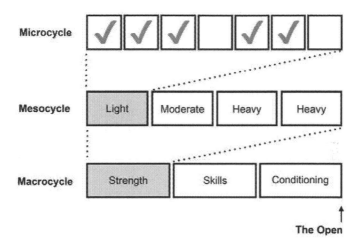

An Example of Periodization in CrossFit

Periodization is a useful tool to create a long-term plan for improvement. By breaking down the training year into smaller parts, your training becomes more focused. This is especially important for skill and strength development, which demands structured training approaches over longer periods of time.

How to use the five principles

Taken together, these five principles of training provide us with practical applications:

- **Use it or lose it.** Do not let too long pass between training the things you want to improve. If you want to increase strength, conditioning, and skills, you should train all three frequently.

- **Manage your training load.** Some of you will want to go to the box almost every day, while others just a few times per week. Fewer sessions can work well with high volume and intensity in each session. In contrast, more sessions mean that your volume or intensity in each session needs to be lower.

- **Vary your training.** Use Metcons to tax all three energy systems regularly. Lift weights over a wide range of intensities, not just as heavy as possible. And practice skills both regularly and consistently, because they require less rest.

- **Create milestones.** Use periodization and cycles to create milestones and specific goals with shorter time frames (a few weeks) in addition to the one big annual goal (the Open).

Chapter 5: Consistency

Knowing what to train for and understanding a few key principles might seem enough to quit reading and start training. But we still haven't discussed the areas most commonly overlooked by athletes who are new to CrossFit. These are injury-preventing strategies, warm-up work, and mobility work.

Ignoring these topics will eventually result in a serious setback, most commonly in the form of mental exhaustion or injury. This not only will prevent you from getting better but can also undo the progress you have made so far.

I have met more athletes—now mostly former athletes—who have ignored these elements than I care to think about. Do not make the same mistake. Being able to keep on training over the long-term is the foundation for progress.

Preventing injury

All movement elevates risk of injury. On the opposite end, lack of movement elevates risk of disease. Both injury and disease endanger your health. But in the developed world, disease is a bigger problem than injuries by an order of magnitude.[1] So although some people refrain from athletic activities because of injury risks, they ignore the fact that any increase in the risk of injury from training will be more than offset by a decrease in the risk of disease.

Although training is good for overall health, you should still strive to minimize your risk of injury. The best way to do this is to choose a sport that gives you large health benefits with few injury risks. This is one of the reasons I was attracted to CrossFit. Compared with other sports, the fitness improvement is high and the injury risk low.

CrossFit is generally safer because it avoids the two most common sources of sports injury. First, there are no tackles or other types of impacts with other athletes. This is the leading cause of injury in popular sports such as basketball, football, and soccer. Second, movements are both varied and short in duration, reducing the risk

1 According to data from the Centers for Disease Control and Prevention, 613 in 100,000 Americans died from the most common diseases in 2014. In comparison, 43 in 100,000 died from accidents. Thus, the average American is at least 14 times more likely to die from disease than an accident. Data: https://www.cdc.gov/ nchs/nvss/mortality/lcwk9.htm

of overuse injuries. These injuries are more common in sports such as long-distance running and track & field.

However, CrossFit is performed at a high intensity. This means that some injury risk is unavoidable. Fitness cannot be increased effectively without risking injury in the process. Fortunately, this risk can be managed. If you plan to do CrossFit for a long time, reducing injury risk should be one of your top priorities.

This goal of reducing injury risk is not only for health reasons but also for performance. Injury is not the end of the world. The human body has an amazing capability to heal. It can recover fully from serious injuries such as torn ligaments, broken bones, and ruptured discs. So most likely, any injury you might sustain during training will be reversible. However, recovery can take a long time and a lot of work. And it will undermine your progress in the meantime.

Marginal improvements in your fitness level matter little if you spend months reverting back to your base level while injured. For sustained progress, your priority should be to reduce the risk of long training-free periods. Only then should you think about improving faster between sessions.

There are some regulars in my box who have stopped improving and only want to maintain their current fitness level. I have asked these few athletes why they are not competing or aiming for more than showing up for WODs. Most of the time, the reason is some injury they sustained during training: "I tore my hamstring," "I dislocated my shoulder," "My Achilles' snapped," or "I think I fractured a disc in my back once." Most of these regulars have recovered either partially or fully, but initially they couldn't train for months. This caused them to lose much of the fitness they had built up over a long time.

Curiously, those I have spoken to all regret something about how they approached the workout when they injured themselves. The three most common regrets I hear are: 1) too heavy lifting at the cost of form, 2) a lack of proper warm-up, and 3) a lack of adequate mobility. All three issues can be prevented if you are smart about your training.

Limit your weights

The following two scenarios are an all-too-common sight at my box, particularly for men. The first is in the weightlifting area, and the second is in Metcons.

1. **Beginners or early intermediates pushing their 1 RMs every week.** Their attempts often result in missed reps and compromised technique, ingraining poor motor patterns and risking injury.

2. **Relative newcomers using too heavy Metcon weights.** These athletes do the workouts too slowly and with poor form. Straight afterward, they rush to the Whiteboard to showcase that they "RX'd" the workout.

If you are guilty of either, please stop and leave your pride outside the box. Stop pushing for personal records if your technique is not solid and you keep missing weights. Failing a lift multiple times will ingrain poor motor patterns and make it more difficult for you to progress. And don't use weights in a Metcon that slow you down to turtle speed and compromise form, just to tick the "RX" mark.

Reduce your 1 RM attempts

A good solution to the first scenario is to mix up your weightlifting intensities by varying the number of repetitions in each set. This reduces your risk of injury during the heaviest lifts. Additionally, it allows you to train more often and with greater volume without overtaxing your body. Finally, it will result in good technique and form, as you will ingrain better technique than with the single lifts. All these benefits translate to greater improvements in the long-term.

However, it is still useful to track performance over time. A good tool for doing this is to use 1 rep max equivalents. This allows you to translate sets with different repetitions into a single scale—the 1 rep max (1 RM). For example, if you train the same lift twice—once with sets of 5 reps and the second time with sets of 8 reps—you can translate both weights into 1 rep max equivalents to compare your sessions or choose appropriate weights.

The most common way to do this is with the Brzycki formula. Named after its creator Matt Brzycki, this formula converts a weight lifted for any number of repetitions into its 1 rep max equivalent. Here is the formula:

1 RM = weight × (36 / (37 - reps))

In order to make it easier for you to make the conversions, I have included a table with the formula used to convert any weight into the different rep schemes. Don't use it for more than 10 reps though, as the formula becomes less accurate as the rep number increases.

Reps	% of 1RM	Weight x __ = 1RM
1	100%	1.00
2	97%	1.03
3	94%	1.06
4	92%	1.09
5	89%	1.13
6	86%	1.16

7	83%	1.20
8	81%	1.24
9	78%	1.29
10	75%	1.33

To illustrate, let's say you are training the back squat. You can currently lift 300 lb. for 3 reps. This means your 1 RM is 300 lb. x (36 / (37 - 3)), or 300 lb. x 1.06 = 318 lb. Instead of pushing to lift 330 lb. once in the next set for a personal record (PR), you could instead lift the same weight again, but for 4 reps. This would also be a PR, since your new 1 RM is now 300 lb. x 1.09 = 327 lb.

In both cases the 1 rep max equivalent has increased. The difference is that your form will be better with the second approach. This helps you ingrain high-quality movement patterns and lowers your risk of injury.

In addition to smarter rep schemes for weightlifting, proper warm-up and mobilization will also reduce injury risk. Including these in your training is essential and should never be overlooked. Additionally, these components not only reduce injury risk but also increase your performance. So instead of just covering them in the context of injuries, we will specifically go over the benefits of and ideal approach to each.

Warming up

If you train at a box and your workouts consist of preprogrammed WODs, then you most likely already warm up at the beginning of each workout. But too often, the warm-up is given little thought. Having dropped in at quite a few boxes, I have found that many warm-up routines are inadequate.

Additionally, many athletes all but ignore them, warming up at the lowest intensity to "save their energy" for the WOD. This makes even the well-designed warm-up routines ineffective.

This neglect of the warm-up becomes most obvious when novice and intermediate athletes work out on their own instead of in class. Some athletes walk into the box, go straight to the barbell, swing it through a few motions, and immediately start piling on the weights.

The underlying assumption behind this behavior is that the warm-up is less important than the actual workout. This is far from the truth. Warming up properly should be an integral part of every workout. In fact, it is so important that if you have limited time, you should skip all the other workout components before removing the critical parts of your warm-up routine.

There are two reasons to develop a good warm-up routine: better performance and lower risk of injury. As staying injury-free is the only way to train consistently, warming up is in essence only about increasing performance. It will help you on the day of training and also ensure you can train again.

How should you warm up?

Having established that we should indeed warm up, let's take a closer look at how to do it properly. A good warm-up routine achieves four things:

1. **Improved circulation.** At rest, your muscles receive only 15–20 percent of their potential blood flow. A full-body warm-up for a few minutes increases this blood flow and opens up the small blood vessels.

2. **Higher body and muscle temperature.** This causes your blood to release more oxygen. It also improves nerve transmissions and muscle metabolism, contributing to increased performance.

3. **Increased range of motion.** This allows you to perform movements with better form, increasing efficiency and safety.

4. **Strengthened movement patterns.** Priming and practicing the movements of the day improves technique. Break down the day's workout into simpler movements with lighter loads. This applies especially to weightlifting and gymnastics, in which good technique is crucial.

Until only 10 to 20 years ago, most athletes warmed up with static stretching, followed by light exercise (jogging, running, biking, and/or rowing). This was ineffective because it didn't meet the goals we've just defined. Additionally, static stretching for 60 seconds or more actually decreases strength in the affected muscles for one to two hours afterward. Thus, while better than not warming up at all, this routine still left much to be desired.

The three essential components

An effective warm-up routine should at minimum contain three components: dynamic stretching, movement circuits, and skill work.

Dynamic stretching is the use of repeated momentum or body positioning to gradually stretch tight muscles into their full range of motion. One example would be swinging a straight leg forward and backward repeatedly, going a little bit higher each time. Another example would be going into a push-up position, bringing one foot forward to the outside of the hand, and moving around in the position to stretch the hips and hamstrings.

These examples are likely familiar to you. In recent years, sports science has demonstrated the benefits of dynamic stretching for warming up. CrossFit has embraced this trend by recommending such exercises for warm-up routines. Dynamic stretches are popular in boxes and are typically selected based on the muscle groups that will be used most in the workout.

The second component is **movement circuits**. In a movement circuit, the athlete goes through a set of full-body functional movements, raising body temperature and improving circulation. The movements are kept similar or the same as movements in the upcoming workout. So if the workout includes burpees and kettlebell swings, an example movement circuit would be 4 rounds of 5 burpees and 10 kettlebell swings with a lower weight.

Movement circuits replace light general exercise with movements related to the activity at hand. This primes good motor patterns and makes sure your muscles are prepared to tackle the workout.

Finally, the third component is **skill work**. Its purpose is to establish solid motor patterns for complex and demanding movements. For weightlifting, this is usually done with a barbell without plates. The athlete focuses on good positions and movement paths. For gymnastics, this entails progressing from simpler movements to the full version required in the workout. For simpler movements, this would mean going through them a few times to practice them with good form. Skill work further strengthens technique and efficiency in the movements to be performed.

Combined, these three components could take anywhere from 15 to 45 minutes, depending on the activity at hand. If you are stiff or sore, or if the workout ahead is intense or complex, go with the higher end of that range. But no matter what the WOD looks like, always include these components in your warm-up.

Other elements to consider

You don't need to limit yourself to only these three components for your warm-up. Many athletes include other elements as well. Here are a few things you can consider adding to your warm-up routine:

- **Foam rolling.** If you are stiff in certain areas, foam rolling can improve circulation and help you loosen up. Be careful to keep this light and save any intense or painful work for later, so it doesn't interfere with your workout.

- **Light exercise.** Running, air biking, rowing, and using the SkiErg can all be effective warm-up exercises. This is especially true if you are sore in muscle groups worked by these exercises. Light exercise to improve circulation in those areas will help you feel more ready to tackle a workout.

- **Breathing exercises.** These are becoming popular and are recommended by coaches of many elite athletes. The idea is to prime the body for movement by improving oxygen uptake and delivery into the muscles. The most common exercise is to practice diaphragmatic breathing while lying on your back.

- **Crossover Symmetry.** This trademarked system uses stretch band exercises to activate the shoulders before a workout. Some athletes find it helpful to remove stiffness or discomfort in the shoulders and shoulder blades. Many boxes have Crossover Symmetry as part of their equipment.

I encourage you to try these additional components to see if they make your warm-up routine more effective.

Cooling down

While not as essential as warming up, a well thought out cool-down routine will aid your training. As you progress to higher levels of performance, this part becomes more important. A cool-down provides you with two main benefits:

- **Enhanced recovery.** Maintaining blood circulation after an intense workout improves recovery. It helps the body flush metabolic waste products out of the muscle cells.

- **Increased flexibility.** Your muscles are warm immediately after a workout. This makes it both easier and safer to stretch them, maintaining or improving your range of motion. Additionally, using a foam roller or massage balls can prevent knots from forming in overworked muscles. This helps you stay flexible for your next workout.

So after your next workout, don't crash to the floor, use the foam roller as a pillow for a few minutes while chatting, and then hit the showers. Instead, consider doing the following:

- **Light exercise.** Stay active for a few minutes, letting your heart rate slowly return to normal. Some good choices are rowing, jogging, biking, and jumping rope.

- **Foam rolling.** Since the workout is finished, you can foam roll specific areas more intensely where you want to reduce stiffness or prevent knots from forming. Try using mobility tools covering a smaller surface area, such as a lacrosse ball.

- **Stretching.** Both active and static stretching can be incorporated into your cool-down routine. Active stretching will increase blood flow to your muscles and maintain your active range of motion. Static stretching will help you increase your flexibility.

CrossFit differs from other sports because the intensity is high in almost every workout. This has clear benefits for your fitness level, but at the same time, it requires you to incorporate proper warm-up and cool-down routines into your workouts. If your box does not incorporate these elements into WODs properly, just show up earlier and stay a bit longer. In the end, you are responsible for your own health and progress, not your coach, so take every step necessary to ensure the best outcome.

Mobilizing

Mobility restrictions are often the biggest hindrance for CrossFit athletes. Without adequate mobility, you spend an excess amount of energy trying to break through these limitations. Your muscles cannot exert their full power, and your mechanics are poor, making movement inefficient.

On top of this, mobility issues multiply your risk of injury. They lead to compensation through poor form, which creates forces that your muscles and joints are not designed to handle.

Despite the negative consequences of mobility restrictions, mobilization is underused. One of the reasons is "paralysis by analysis." There is so much advice on how we should mobilize that it becomes overwhelming. Consequently, many athletes lack clear mobilization goals, instead stretching randomly for a few minutes after each workout and calling it a day.

This behavior stems from a lack of understanding of the principles beneath all this mobilization advice. Without such an understanding, the advice becomes confusing and difficult to follow.

The main source of this confusion is that mobilization expertise is fragmented. Most experts in the field specialize in one particular method that is presented to you as the best solution, when another method might actually be more appropriate to resolve your issue.

An old proverb captures this concept well: if all you have is a hammer, everything looks like a nail. So, for example, going to a chiropractor with your problem will result in joint manipulations to resolve it. Going with the same problem to a sports massage therapist will result in soft tissue work. And going to a medical doctor might result in prescribed medication.

The lesson is that you cannot outsource your mobility to experts. You are the only person who can determine which method works best for your specific problem.

Before we even get into details, however, be clear on what your goal is. Why do you want to use mobilization techniques? Just because you are told to do so and everyone else seems to be doing them? Or are you trying to achieve a specific goal? To answer this, let's take a look at the objectives of mobilization and whether you think they are beneficial for you.

Full mobility doesn't exist

As can be derived from the word, the goal of mobilization is *mobility*. In the context of physiology, mobility is the ability to move one's body through physical space. We all have this ability but to varying degrees. A couch potato with no exercise background will be less mobile than an elite gymnast, to take two examples.

In this book, we define mobility specifically in the context of CrossFit. We refer to full mobility as the ability to perform every CrossFit movement effectively through a full range of motion. By "effectively," we mean without any hindrance such as tightness, pain, loss of form, or loss of power. By this definition, an athlete who meets this criterion for all movements is considered to be fully mobile. So, if you can perform every CrossFit movement without issue, you can consider yourself fully mobile.

Full mobility is the ultimate goal of all mobilization work. But in reality, no athlete can be considered fully mobile. Everyone benefits from improving something, be it more ankle range of motion, less hip resistance when squatting, decreased stiffness in the shoulders, or a number of other things. Thus, you will never actually reach your goal of full mobility. But by working toward it, you can move closer to this ideal each day.

Keeping this in mind simplifies mobilization work. Knowing that the journey is endless relieves you of perfectionistic tendencies when it comes to implementation. Your aim suddenly becomes simple:

increase your mobility just a little bit more than before the session.

Get the biggest bang for your buck

Mobilization is neither complicated nor overwhelming. Granted, you can always dig deeper when it comes to specific issues, areas, or techniques. But the ultimate purpose is simple: to allow you to perform the CrossFit movements better.

By knowing this, you can approach mobilization more practically. It is just a matter of following a few logical steps. The first is identifying your mobility restrictions. The second is prioritizing them. And the third is resolving them with the techniques you find most effective.

1. Identify your mobility restrictions

Your first step is to identify which mobility restrictions you have. You've probably already started such a list in your head. You might have an area of tightness. Some movements or positions may cause you discomfort. You might lack the flexibility for a full range of motion with certain movements. Some muscles might be constantly stiff. A particular joint may be impaired. All things like this that bother you should be on your list.

If you already have a list like this clear in your head, you don't need to do anything more in this first step. Just keep it simple and move to the next step. You can always come back to the identification step once you have resolved your most pressing issues.

But if you are unsure of which restrictions you have, you can perform a quick self-diagnostic. Take a PVC pipe, or a broomstick if you are at home, and perform an overhead squat. The overhead squat is the best diagnostic tool when it comes to mobility issues. Both the beginning and end positions reveal many issues you may have with the most common CrossFit movements.

Have someone film you or film yourself in these positions and aim to answer the following questions with a yes. If you cannot do so, the reason is most likely a mobility issue.

- **Ankles:** Do they have the required range of motion?
- **Knees:** Do they bend smoothly through the full range of motion? Are they aligned with your toes?
- **Hips:** Can you sit in the bottom position with the weight centered in the front part of your heels?
- **Hip flexors:** Is your spine neutral in the starting position?
- **Spine:** Can you maintain a neutral position in both starting and end positions?
- **Lats:** Are your elbows fully extended in the beginning position?

- **Shoulders:** Do your shoulders stay in good position? Is the pipe or broomstick over your heels? Are your arms behind your ears?

- **Wrists:** Can you comfortably hold the pipe or broomstick?

Performing this self-diagnostic will help you create a list of mobility issues that you would like to fix. If you want to learn about proper body mechanics and identifying issues in more detail, I have recommended some resources at the end of the chapter.

2. Prioritize your list

Which restrictions are holding your performance back the most? Which bother you because of pain or discomfort? And which are causing the greatest risk of injury by compromising your form? Let these questions guide you to order the list you have made. And start with the most pressing issue at the top of the list.

3. Resolve the issues, one by one

With this list in hand (or in mind), you are now ready to take a structured, effects-based approach to improving your mobility. Start with your highest-priority restriction and experiment with ways to resolve it.

Only now do different mobility techniques come into play. Try some different methods you think are likely to help, and evaluate the results. Essentially, you are taking the role of a scientist, experimenting with different methods and seeing what works best. To give you a starting point, here is a list of common mobility techniques you can consider. Some we have already discussed, others not:

- **Chiropractic:** Joint manipulation through controlled introduction of a rapid force. This results in a "popping" sound as gas bubbles in the joint break down.

- **Dynamic stretching:** Use of repeated momentum or body positioning to gradually stretch tight muscles into their full range of motion. For example, swinging a straight leg forward and backward repeatedly, going a little bit higher each time.

- **Foam rolling:** Concentrated stretching of soft tissues. Foam rolls, lacrosse balls, and other methods of releasing "trigger points" fall into this category. The technical term for this technique is *myofascial release*.

- **Massage:** Similar to foam rolling but focuses more on repeated rubbing and kneading of the soft tissues.

- **Muscle activation:** Light exercises that activate and strengthen muscles to increase stability and range of motion.

- **Posture diagnosis:** Inspection of posture and movement patterns to identify form breakdown, contributing to mobility issues.

- **Repeat stretching:** Repeatedly stretching the muscle for a few seconds, contracting it for a few seconds, and then relaxing further into the stretch. The technical term is *PNF (proprioceptive neuromuscular facilitation) stretching.*

- **Static stretching:** Stretching of muscles with the body at rest, usually for at least 30–60 seconds per stretch.

Using these techniques, try to resolve your most limiting mobility restriction. Once you have improved adequately, move on to the next restriction on your list. By continually experimenting like this, you will develop increased knowledge and self-awareness when it comes to your mobility, allowing you to solve future issues more effectively.

Mobility resources

There are a few main resources I use to learn how to improve my mobility. I have listed them here if you want to educate yourself further:

- *Becoming a Supple Leopard:* Written by mobilization pioneer Kelly Starrett, this book provides a wide range of tools for self-diagnosis and improving your mobility. It includes positional analysis, movement corrections, and hundreds of mobilization techniques. It also includes a program for each body part if you want to focus on a certain area. This book is one of the best mobilization resources in my view.

- **MobilityWOD.com:** This website is another project of Kelly Starrett, only here the teaching is through videos instead of text and photos. You can follow daily mobility programming and learn about the same topics as in the book.

- **ROMWOD.com:** This is a daily yoga-like program but with more focus on positions that aid you in CrossFit movements. You can select the daily workout or specific exercises based on problem areas. I try to do this daily to keep myself mobile.

- **Websites and videos:** Often, I have found the best advice by searching online for the specific issue I have at hand. There are countless websites, blogs, videos, and articles providing advice on all kinds of mobility issues. Sometimes, techniques from such online resources have helped me the most.

These resources have helped me identify techniques that work well for my specific restrictions. The good thing about mobilization techniques is that they are harmless most of the time. This allows you to safely try out a lot of things and see what works best. I encourage you to go on a journey to tackle your mobility restrictions consistently. You will reap the benefits both in workouts and in your overall wellness.

Chapter 6: Workouts

Now that we've covered the background information required for training effectively, we can get into the actual workouts. We will look at the three key competencies that Open workouts demand: skills, strength, and conditioning.

As you read in the first part, these are the areas you should focus on. For each, we will discuss the most effective way to improve. At the end of this chapter, we will also review the most common training equipment.

Skills

Skill level, or technique, is all about performing a movement efficiently. In some cases, your skill level will determine whether you can perform the movement at all. Thus, your skill level, not just your strength and conditioning, will dictate your results in many workouts.

We all recognize the importance of skills when it comes to certain movements. Some athletes cannot string together large numbers of double-unders. Others have a hard time with the muscle-up. Still others struggle with technique in the Olympic lifts. All these problems come down to a lack of skills.

But there are more movements with a strong skill component. Handstand push-ups, for instance, improve rapidly once you start practicing them. The same is true for push jerks, toes-to-bars, and pull-ups. These movements have a strong neurological component. By practicing them consistently with good form, we ingrain them in our "muscle memory" and can perform them better the next time around.

There is a seemingly endless set of skills that you could spend your time developing. The kip, butterflies, handstands, Olympic lifts, toes-to-bars, accessory lifts, double-unders. What should you focus on? How frequently should you do it? And how much time should you devote to skill training?

A lack of good guidelines for skill improvement leads to many athletes just sticking to WODs. They hope that this will develop their skill levels over time. This is ineffective for two reasons. First, WODs are usually centered on weightlifting and Metcons. This means that dedicated skill practice is largely omitted. Second, the constant variation of WODs means that your skill training will be sporadic. As we will see, this is not conducive to learning.

The importance of consistent practice

The most important factor when it comes to skill improvement is *consistent practice*. A good example of this principle is musicians improving their instrument skills. Everyone who is serious about mastering an instrument is taught to practice, even just for a little bit, every single day.

Playing an instrument is a neurological skill. You have to learn coordination and proper movements of many muscles in harmony. This is best developed with so-called repetitive reinforcement. You practice every day so you don't forget, consciously or subconsciously, what you learned from the previous session. This enables you to keep building on top of your current level.

Another advantage of daily practice is how quickly you accumulate practice time. If you practice consistently, the best indicator of your skill level is *the total time spent practicing the specific skill*. To illustrate, consider three possible scenarios for an athlete trying to improve a certain movement skill: daily practice for 5 minutes, weekly practice of 20 minutes (i.e., skill work after a weekend WOD), and practice every other week for 1 hour (a dedicated skill workout).

Frequency of practice	Time per session	Time per month	Sessions per month
Daily	5 minutes	2.5 hours	30 sessions
Weekly	20 minutes	2 hours	4 sessions
Monthly	1 hour	1 hour	1 session

The results that stand out are from daily skill work, even for only five minutes. Not only do you accumulate the greatest amount of time training, but the total number of sessions is by far the highest. This means that you will continually build on top of your current skill level instead of partially forgetting what you learned in the previous session.

In fact, if you stick to a low frequency of skill training, you may never progress further than your current skill level. You will only maintain your current level in most movements.

These facts provide you with an opportunity. With consistent skill practice, you will soon surpass other athletes in demanding movements. Now all you need are the right ingredients for your plan—which skills to focus on, when, and for how long.

Focus on the essentials

To identify the most important skills to focus on, we will revisit the chart from chapter 1 that shows the most common Open movements. Only this time, we will categorize them by the limiting factor to performance—skill, strength, or conditioning.

Some movements are limited primarily by your strength or conditioning. You improve these by training at high intensity. Training these movements with high loads and/or repetitions under stress builds up your work capacity.

Other movements have a larger skill component. You improve these best by practicing frequently at lower intensity. This way, you ingrain the movement patterns with frequent exposure but without the need for long recovery.

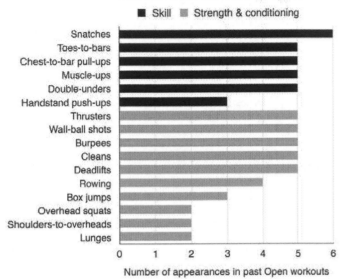

Workout Movements by Type

■ Skill   ▨ Strength & conditioning

Number of appearances in past Open workouts

Note: Different variations of similar movements are grouped together for simplicity. This includes the power and squat variations of snatches and cleans, ring muscle-ups and bar muscle-ups, and dumbbell and barbell variations of lunges, cleans, and snatches.

The breakdown in this chart reveals that six Open movements have a large skill component: snatches, toes-to-bars, chest-to-bar pull-ups, muscle-ups, double-unders, and handstand push-ups.

Mastering these six movements should be your number one priority when it comes to skill training. It might be fun to practice the butterfly technique or free handstands, but it will be of little use when it comes to the Open. If you want to become a better Open athlete, focus your skill training on these six movements.

A disclaimer is in order. All models are inaccurate by design, as they oversimplify reality. Grouping the Open movements in this way is one such model, used to gain a specific insight. Many of the skill-based movements have a strong strength component as well. For example, a newcomer to CrossFit will need to build up strength in addition to skill to complete high-repetition sets of handstand push-ups.

On the other side of the coin, the strength and conditioning movements also have a skill component. Burpees are very taxing when you haven't performed them in a long time, but they become easier if you do them frequently. This difference is because your nervous system adapts to these movement just like your muscles do. So make sure not to ignore the other movements.

That being said, your handstand push-ups will improve faster with daily practice than with weekly high-rep workouts. Conversely, doing burpees daily is unnecessary. Only one session per week, such as in a WOD, would be enough to perform them efficiently when called upon.

Know where you stand

A good start for dedicated skill training is to find out your current level for each movement. Can you string together 50–100 double-unders? What about 10–20 handstand push-ups? With questions like these, comparing yourself to others in your box will probably give you a rough estimate of where you stand.

For a better estimate, I have listed here some key benchmarks. They can help you determine when you have reached an adequate skill level in each movement. An adequate level translates to the movement not being a bottleneck in an Open workout, allowing you to focus on other things.

- **Muscle-ups:** 10 unbroken, both in the rings and on the bar
- **Double-unders:** 100 unbroken
- **Snatches:** 1.25 x body weight
- **Toes-to-bars:** 15 unbroken
- **Chest-to-bar pull-ups:** 30 unbroken
- **Handstand push-ups:** 20 unbroken

If you can reach this level for a movement, consider yourself "graduated" and move on to the next one. If you are not there yet, aim to achieve a similar level in all movements to eliminate weaknesses.

If you manage to train all movements to your desired level, set up a schedule to maintain your skills. Your performance will deteriorate if you don't practice the movements regularly.

For an even more thorough analysis, I recommend the website Beyond the Whiteboard (beyondthewhiteboard .com). There, you can see how your performance in every movement compares to tens of thousands of other athletes. For example, you could insert your max reps for the handstand push-ups and see your percentile ranking. This way, you can accurately identify your strengths and weaknesses.

Start improving

Now, your skill weaknesses should be clear. Start practicing daily the movement you are the weakest at. To make the plan realistic, you can limit it to workout days and a very short time. For instance, if your biggest weakness is double-unders, devote five minutes after each workout to practice.

I will not get into detailed advice on how to specifically improve each of the six movements we've discussed. Specifics for training all of them can be found for free by searching online. Generally, the best way to learn a specific movement, aside from coaching, is to watch a demonstration video and then practice what you have seen. Additionally, here are some tips to make your skill training effective:

- **Practice around your WOD.** To make things practical, add skill training to your existing WODs. Spend five minutes before or after a workout to practice a specific skill as a part of your warm-up or cool-down. Some skills, like double-unders, are well suited to train in this way.

- **Measure your progress.** When you start practicing a skill, make sure you log your current level. For example, if you want to improve your double-unders, write down your current biggest set, smallest set, and average set. As the numbers improve, you will be motivated to continue.

- **Film yourself.** The skill-based movements depend on positioning your body correctly. Most beginners lack the kinetic self-awareness to do so. By filming yourself and comparing to correct form, you gain valuable visual feedback. Use it to improve your technique, internalizing what good movement feels like.

- **Use progressions.** If you cannot perform a movement, use easier variations at first and gradually transition to the full version. This method is called a progression. There are plenty of freely available progressions for every movement online.

- **Don't overspecialize.** Once you are good enough in a movement, move on to the next one. It can be tempting to continue focusing on double-unders once you can manage an unbroken set of 100. But by that time, you are better served learning a skill that needs developing.

Strength

Strength training is more prominent in WODs than skill training, so it requires less introduction. But in both areas, progress demands a structured approach.

The key difference between the two is the time frame. While you can improve skills with a week of daily training sessions, the same will not work for strength. After an intense weightlifting session, the body adapts by changing muscle tissues, bones, and ligaments. This adaptation demands a longer recovery time than neural adaptations to skill training.

This attribute of strength development has caused frustration for many athletes. For the beginner, there are no problems at first. In fact, for the first 6–12 months, personal records seem to fall almost every time you pick up the barbell. But after this initial adaptation period, the body becomes acclimated to the load. As a result, progress slows or even stops completely. This is the much-dreaded plateau many of us have encountered.

For those who want to excel in the Open, riding out this wave of initial strength increases will not be adequate. As we have seen, a third of Open workouts will test your strength. An athlete who has followed an effective strength program will be rewarded on the Leaderboard in those workouts.

The three types of strength

Strength development can seem complex and difficult to understand. However, we can focus our approach by looking at previous weightlifting movements in the Open. When we categorize them according to the type of strength required, a simpler pattern emerges.

The following table shows a breakdown of every Open movement from the last five years according to the type of strength required. Here, I count the frequency of each movement appearing in a workout in the past and add those together for each type of strength.

Movement	Fre-quency	Pull-ing?	Squat-ting?	Press-ing?
Snatches	6	Yes	Yes	Yes
Cleans	5	Yes	Yes	
Thrusters	5		Yes	Yes
Deadlifts	5	Yes		
Overhead squats	2		Yes	Yes
Shoulders-to-over-heads	2			Yes
Lunges	2		Yes	
Total frequency		**16**	**20**	**15**

From this, we can see that Open workouts test three primary types of strength:

- **Pulling.** Picking up an object from the ground using the posterior chain (i.e., the back, glutes, hamstrings, lats, and traps). The movements that require pulling strength are snatches, cleans, and deadlifts.

- **Squatting.** Lifting an object using our hips and knees. These movements are snatches, cleans, thrusters, overhead squats, and lunges.

- **Pressing.** Moving an object over our heads. These movements are snatches, thrusters, overhead squats, and shoulders-to-overheads (moving an object from shoulder height to the overhead position).

These three main types of strength are relatively equal when it comes to frequency of appearance. Therefore, to prepare for the Open, we should simultaneously focus on developing pulling, squatting, and pressing strength.

If you focus on these three strength types, all weightlifting movements you encounter will become easier. For example, if you improve your clean, your deadlift will improve as well, as both movements rely heavily on your pulling strength.

This insight makes strength training easier to implement, as we only need to track three elements instead of every single weightlifting movement. By tracking how often you are training these three types, you will get a good overview of your strength development progress.

Practical strategies

A few additional tips for strength training:

- **Get feedback on technique.** As you progress, the weights involved become heavier. Good technique is paramount to reducing the risk of injury and ensuring you activate the right muscle groups. Ideally, this will be in the form of coaching from an experienced weightlifting coach. Additionally, get visual feedback by recording and watching your lifts. You can compare them with videos of the best athletes to see what you need to improve.

- **Use a variety of loads.** As we covered in the Principles chapter, strength development is most effective when you expose yourself to a variety of loads. That means you shouldn't fixate only on lifting weights at 80–100 percent of your 1 rep max but also in the lower-intensity ranges. This has the added benefit of reducing injury risk and allowing you to increase training volume.

- **Optimize the training load.** Ensure optimal loads on the three types of strength. This will maintain the highest rate of improvement. Also make sure you don't ignore any of the three types for prolonged periods of time. Only back squatting for strength will undermine your pulling and pressing ability over time.

- **Educate yourself.** The sports of weightlifting and Olympic lifting have been around for longer than CrossFit. Take advantage of this and educate yourself on the underlying principles. There are great resources available in both fields.

Key benchmarks

Here are some benchmarks for the key lifts. You can use these to determine where you stand and identify strengths and weaknesses. If you have reached the benchmark for one of these lifts, move on and focus on the benchmarks you haven't reached yet.

- **Back squat:** 2 x body weight
- **Front squat:** 1.8 x body weight
- **Overhead squat:** 1 x body weight
- **Deadlift:** 3 x body weight
- **Snatch:** 1.25 x body weight
- **Clean & jerk:** 1.5 x body weight

Conditioning

Conditioning is the great separator in the sport of CrossFit. While skills and strength are important attributes, conditioning will ultimately determine your place on the Leaderboard. And what exactly is conditioning? Simply put, it is our ability to deliver *power*—as much work as possible in the shortest time possible.

As we saw in chapter 1, the Open is primarily a test of conditioning. Every single workout in the last five years of the competition has tested this ability. No matter which workout you look at, the goal is always to get the most work done in the least amount of time. This is the essence of CrossFit. While strength and skills are necessary tools, the real test is how fast you can put them to use.

Conditioning can be broken down into two attributes: metabolic conditioning (which Metcons derive their name from) and muscular endurance. The former is a measure of how effectively our energy systems can deliver power, and the latter is a measure of how well our strength translates into higher-repetition workouts. The two are closely related and often trained simultaneously.

While skill training requires a short recovery period and strength training longer, conditioning is somewhere in between. Low-intensity conditioning sessions require little time to recover from and can even aid recovery. Conversely, the most intense sessions can take as long to recover from as maximum-effort strength workouts.

Conditioning is not a one-dimensional skill of pushing yourself harder and "grinding it out." As your experience increases, you develop various abilities that increase your power output. Examples include pacing, breaking down large sets of a movement, moving smoothly, transitioning quickly, optimizing pause durations, maintaining effective breathing, and ignoring the discomfort that urges you to quit or slow down.

You develop these abilities with repeated exposure to conditioning workouts over a long period of time. In this way, conditioning development shares many of the same principles as the skills development we discussed earlier. In order to improve your conditioning, you need to expose yourself regularly to these kinds of workouts. If you don't, you enter a detraining phase in which your conditioning gradually declines.

Practical performance tips

- **Include aerobic work.** In general, high-intensity interval training (HIIT) is more effective to develop conditioning than is longer-duration aerobic work. However, our aerobic energy system is used extensively in all workouts as well. Training the aerobic system creates adaptations that allow you to push harder in the shorter time domains. Experiment with running, rowing, swimming, and/or cycling at an easy pace for 40–60 minutes. It will help you sustain a higher power output in shorter workouts.

- **"Train slower to race faster."** In Metcons, you likely push yourself to the highest intensity, trying to get a better placement on the Whiteboard than your peers. This will limit the amount of volume you can achieve and can also increase your risk of injury. Mixing in training at lower intensities will allow you to train more often.[1]

- **Use progressions.** Just as with skills and weightlifting, you can use progressions to develop conditioning. For example, schedule an interval session each week that becomes more difficult over time. Your body will progressively adapt to the greater load, just like with weightlifting. This will let you achieve conditioning levels higher than you would get only with randomized Metcons.

---

1 This principle was largely popularized by Clyde Hart. He was the coach of Michael Johnson, one of the most successful track & field runners in history. It has since spread to other fields, including distance running, martial arts, and weightlifting. You can read an interview with Hart about this principle in American Track & Field, Merit Rankings Issue (2005): page 58. The full text is available here: http://richwoodstrack.com/rhs_team_area/sprints/tech_Slow_Train_ClydeHart.pdf

- **Mix in recovery-friendly movements.** One challenge with Metcons is how taxing they can be on the body. A couplet or triplet consisting of barbell work and sprinting, for example, can require a long time to fully recover from. Conversely, movements such as rowing, swimming, and cycling are much less taxing. They don't make your muscles sore through eccentric loading or stress your joints with repeated impact. Take advantage of this for your aerobic work and progressions. It will enable you to train your conditioning without wearing out your muscles and joints and interfering with the rest of your training.

Key benchmarks

When assessing your level of conditioning, be careful not to rely on benchmarks that also test your strength or skill level. If you do so, you cannot attribute progress to your conditioning alone. Instead, use purer tests of conditioning. Here are some benchmarks for a high level of conditioning:

- **500 m row:** 1:30 min. (men) / 1:40 min. (women)
- **2 km row:** 6:40 min. (men) / 7:30 min. (women)
- **1 mile run:** 6 min.
- **5 km run:** 20 min. (men) / 21 min. (women)

MINI-CHAPTER:

Equipment

Personal equipment is not a big factor when it comes to CrossFit performance. I will assume that your box already has the equipment required for all the workouts (bars and bumpers, boxes, jump ropes, etc.) and also the equipment required for mobility work (foam rollers, lacrosse balls, bands, etc.). Thus, I will only cover the equipment bought personally on top of these things.

Shoes

Good shoes are important in CrossFit. Solid heel support ensures stability and increases safety when lifting heavy weights. A factor to consider is the heel drop of your shoes, i.e., the height reduction from the heel to the toes. Shoes with low (2–4 millimeters) or no heel drop are common. However, such a flat sole can impede proper mechanics in the Olympic lifts. Many athletes lack ankle flexibility, resulting in the load shifting forward from the heels into the toes in such situations.

If this is a problem for you, consider a shoe with a heel drop of 8 mm or more. For workouts that only include weightlifting and/or Olympic lifting, you can also consider dedicated Olympic weightlifting shoes. They have a high heel drop, often 20–30 mm. This enables the athlete to remain more upright through squatting movements, reducing shear forces on the back and allowing for less ankle mobility.

Jump rope

Double-unders are one of the most common Open movements. They are largely skill based, so you should be practicing them regularly. By having your own jump rope, you will get used to its feel and length during these practice sessions. This will make your technique more consistent in a workout. The handles are a question of personal preference. But for the wire, I recommend a thin and light version to reduce the load on your shoulders, which keeps the wrists in position as the band circles around you.

The second point to consider: don't cut the rope too short! I have made this mistake more than once. It is always easier to shorten your rope a little bit later. Lengthening, however, usually means you need to buy a new wire.

Grips

Most people rip their palms when doing movements on a bar without grips. If you are one of them, find a grip you like and stick to it. If you use leather, replace the grips regularly when they become stiff and coarse. Otherwise, the grips themselves will start to cause tears.

Knee sleeves

Knee sleeves are mostly for comfort, such as when you lunge on a hard surface. But they are also meant to reduce the risk of injury by keeping the knee joints warm. Some also find them helpful for increased kinetic feedback as the knee moves within the sleeve. However, others find them uncomfortable as the sleeve folds up in the back of the knee when squatting, pushing the joint apart.

Wrist wraps

Wraps can be used to keep the wrists warm and reduce the risk of strains by providing support. This can be nice for burpees, for instance, when you throw yourself quickly to the floor with your wrists absorbing the impact. Many athletes also find them helpful for overhead stability, such as in heavy snatches and jerks. However, wrist wraps can limit strength development in the forearms, eventually making those who wear them regularly weaker without them. So if you do use wraps, limit their use so you don't need to rely on them.

Tape

Tape is mostly used to protect the thumbs from tearing when using the hook grip with heavy weights or high volume. This applies especially to the snatch, where the thumbs have a larger contact area with the bar. If you use it, try to find a tape that doesn't detract from your grip. Also, don't stretch it so tight that it reduces mobility in your thumbs.

Compression clothing

Some wear compression tops, tights, and socks. The idea is to increase blood circulation in the muscles. However, for high repetitions at high intensities, this can be counterproductive. In those cases, compression can limit the ability of the muscles to circulate blood into and out of the muscles, reducing circulation. So, if you want to use compression clothing, limit its use to low-rep weightlifting or low-intensity workouts, such as jogging or biking.

Lifting belt

A lifting belt is used to improve bracing in heavy lifts. When properly used, a belt increases intra-abdominal pressure, which helps your spine stay in a neutral position. Belts are used by most advanced athletes, but for beginners, improving mechanics and mobility is a better strategy. If you are an intermediate, you can try out a belt when squatting/deadlifting (to prevent rounding) and pressing/ jerking (to prevent overextension) and see if it helps you. Just make sure to learn proper bracing. Finally, using a belt for high-rep sets will probably hinder you more than help you because it will reduce your oxygen intake.[1]

---

1 For more detail, CrossFit Invictus has a good article about using lifting belts in the sport. Read it here: https://www.crossfitinvictus.com/blog/what-about-lifting-belts

Chapter 7: Programming

Now you are armed with the fundamental knowledge required to train effectively. The most difficult part, however, is translating this into a practical workout schedule. This task is as much art as science. The factors to consider are simply too many for a definitive solution to exist. Programming is the process of solving this problem.

The programming landscape

Most professional athletes rely on coaches to program for them. This way, they follow personalized training schedules designed by specialists. The advantage of this is that the athlete can focus solely on execution. Long periods of research and experimentation with different approaches are left for the coach to explore.

Personalized coaching is not realistic for most aspiring athletes. Good coaches devote their time to those who are at the top of the sport, staying out of reach for the rest. Additionally, there are other challenges with this approach, such as the cost of personalized coaching and time commitment required to follow it. After adding these to the equation, the possibility of such coaching becomes more remote.

Luckily, aspiring athletes have other options. Although the Web has made programming more confusing than before, it has also made top-tier coaching more accessible. There are now programs from great coaches available online for a low or no monthly fee. These programs sometimes include elements from personal coaching, such as consultations, tailored programming for the individual, and feedback on technique.

However, none of these options eliminates the need for basic knowledge of the fundamentals of programming. This knowledge helps with selecting an effective program that suits your personal needs. Without any knowledge, you can fall prey to well-marketed programs that are actually ineffective given the goals you want to reach. Sooner or later, these programs will leave you frustrated with your lack of progress.

To prevent this, I've provided here the tools you need to make an informed decision on your own programming. As with mobilization, your programming experience will gradually grow as you experiment with what works best. Over time, you will be able to fully guide your own training, knowing what works best for you personally.

When choosing or designing your training schedule, I recommend taking the following five steps:

1. Measure your baseline
2. Define your goals
3. Assess how well your current program meets your goals
4. Research the different options available
5. Choose the right option

These five steps help you clarify your objectives and ensure that the program you choose supports them.

1. Measure your baseline

The first step in programming is to assess your current ability. Most likely, you already do this informally. You have some idea of which aspects of the sport are strengths for you and which are weaknesses. However, this informal assessment has the downside of not being measurable.

To accurately assess your current level of performance, use the key benchmarks for the three domains of fitness—skills, strength, and conditioning—from chapter 6 and write down the results. This will form the baseline for your program.

2. Define your goals

The next part is to define what you want to achieve. This will be your guidance when assessing your current programming and also when choosing from other options.

Consider the following example. Let's say the Open is six months from now and you have just finished the baseline measurement. You have great conditioning according to the benchmarks, but you are lacking in both skills and strength. As we saw in chapter 2, eliminating your weaknesses will give you the biggest boost when it comes to the Open Leaderboard. Keeping that in mind, you define the following goals:

- **Skills:** Reach an intermediate level in all skills within three months. Reach the benchmarks in all skills within six months.

- **Strength:** Reach 80 percent of the benchmark levels in all movements within four months. Then maintain those levels until the Open.

- **Conditioning:** Maintain current level for the next four months. Then emphasize conditioning until the Open starts.

This type of goal setting is well defined, time-specific, and realistic. Knowing that skills improve faster than strength, you aim for bigger improvements in that area. Knowing that you are punished more for your weaknesses than rewarded for your strengths, you focus on increased balance. And knowing that conditioning will be the main test, you aim to maintain your strength and skill improvements while building power until the Open begins.

Go through the same goal-setting exercise after assessing your current level of performance. Equipped with the insights from this book, you will have no trouble setting clearly defined goals in a similar way.

3. Assess your current program

Before choosing a path forward, look back on the path that has led you to the place you are at currently. Continuing with our example, let's assume you have attended WODs in your box four to five times per week for the last year. The baseline shows you the results: the programming in your box has improved your conditioning, but your skills and strength gains are limited.

Your task in this step is to analyze why this has happened. Inspect the workouts you have attended for the last few months and analyze them using the frameworks in this book. How many WODs have included skill development? What about strength and conditioning? And what has been the frequency of each? The following table shows a framework for this analysis along with hypothetical results from our example.

Analysis of Past Workouts

Domain	Subset	Component	Workouts in the last month
Skills	Gymnastics	Muscle-ups	x
		Toes-to-bars	x x x
		Chest-to-bar pull-ups	x
		Handstand push-ups	x
	Conditioning	Double-unders	x x
Weightlifting	Olympic	Snatch	x x
		Clean & jerk	x x
	Strength	Squatting	x x x x x
		Pulling	x x
		Pressing	x x
Conditioning	Metcons	Shorter (< 10 min.)	x x x xx x xx x
		Longer (10–20 min.)	xx x xxx x x x x
	Endurance	Aerobic work	

With this analysis, we can now see the reason for this imbalanced development. Although the training schedule has been consistent, Metcons have been the focus of almost all workouts. Skill work has been sporadic, Olympic lifting sessions few, strength work unbalanced among the three types of strength, and aerobic work ignored. This type of visual analysis will give you a good idea of the changes you need to make.

The deficiencies in your previous programming become glaringly obvious once you go through this analysis. Do not beat yourself up for not realizing this earlier. Instead, consider yourself lucky to finally have these insights now.

Also keep in mind that programming needs are different for different individuals. The WODs you have been attending may have been exactly what the average athlete needs to get healthier. You are simply striving for a more ambitious goal.

4. Research the different options available

Many excellent programming choices exist today. Armed with the knowledge from this book, you are now in a good position to evaluate them based on your needs. But before you choose a specific option, know that there are different routes you can go. Some athletes choose a combination of these options:

- **Real-life personalized coaching.** Generally, the only people who do this are full-time professional athletes or those who want to join them. That's because this option is the costliest in terms of both financial and time requirements. If you go this route, only settle for a coach with a demonstrated track record of developing great athletes. Otherwise, you are likely better served with the other options.

- **Remote personalized coaching.** This option is becoming more popular, particularly among athletes who aim to qualify for Regionals. It is still a big commitment, however, particularly if you heed the same advice as for the first option: settling only for a great coach.

- **360° online programming.** With this option, you receive all your programming from one source. On top of this, you may be provided with instructions on warm-ups, cool-down, mobility, recovery, nutrition, and even lifestyle. These programs are often designed for peak performance at a particular point, such as during the Open, Regionals, or Games. Many top-level athletes choose this option.

- **Partial online programming.** Another option is to add to your current training schedule an online program designed for that purpose. This way, you can add a specific gymnastics, strength, Olympic lifting, or conditioning module, depending on your needs. At the same time, you can keep attending your current program, such as the WODs in your box.

- **Workout of the Day.** For most athletes, the WOD in their box is the program of choice. Almost everyone starts this way, learning to show up and work out consistently. And most stay here for the full duration of their time in the sport. This is the simplest option, as you just have to show up and do what you are told. This is a big benefit if the program in your box is well designed.

- **Your own programming.** The final option is to design your own program. Many competitive athletes do this to some degree. An example would be adding your own progressions to tackle a specific weakness not addressed by your current program.

There are plenty of different programs available within each category. This book will not provide you with such a list, as the list changes rapidly and everyone's needs are different. Instead, do your own research online. I recommend searching CrossFit blogs and online forums for an up-to-date list of options.

5. Choose the right program

Before you choose a program, consider all the implications of the route you want to follow. For example, if you are relatively inexperienced, following an online program can be a poor choice. You may lack adequate technique to perform the key movements with good form. This makes the WOD, where a coach can give you feedback, a better choice. You may also lack the training experience to endure the load. Online programs are often designed for experienced athletes who can train harder than newcomers.

Also, if you want to move away from the WOD in your box, make sure you have the motivation to follow through with it. Having a training partner, for example, may make the transition more sustainable in the long-term.

With all this in mind, the last step—actually selecting what to do—should be the easiest. You already know where you stand and where you want to go. Now it is simply a question of choosing the option that is most likely to get you there in the least amount of time. So make your choice and enjoy the journey ahead.

PART III: RECOVERY

No matter how much you train, most of your hours will be spent recovering. During this time, you will make many decisions that affect how well your body and mind adapt to training.

The speed and effectiveness of recovery depends partially on factors outside of your control. Age, genetics, and training experience are three examples. However, many factors are fully within your control. In this section, we will cover the most relevant ones. They are nutrition, lifestyle, and supplements.

Chapter 8: Nutrition

What you eat has a big effect on both your recovery and performance. Being mindful about the foods you eat can translate to a big advantage in training.

Advice on nutrition has always been fuzzy. Many fad diets have become popular, only to fade away as a new trend rises a few years later. These changes often happen when a celebrity advocates a new diet or through other types of marketing efforts. One of the reasons for this chaos in the nutrition realm is a gap in most people's knowledge of the principles of nutrition.

Principles of a healthy diet

Luckily, these "fashion trends" are becoming less prominent as nutrition science fills up our knowledge gaps. Research has established sound principles that we can follow to improve our performance.

The beneficial effects of following these principles are not limited to training. A healthy diet will improve your mental health and reduce the risks of many diseases, including diabetes, heart disease, and cancer.

Although this chapter focuses on nutrition in the context of CrossFit, we will not ignore these added "side effects." Greater mental health and reduced risk of disease will help you with any effort in the long run.

Without further ado, let's review these principles:

- **Eat whole foods.** These are foods that do not contain labels with lists of ingredients because they are the ingredients themselves. Whole foods are the most nutritious foods you can find. In contrast, processed foods have fewer nutrients but more calories, a combination that harms your health.

- **Avoid processed foods.** Contrary to whole foods, many processed foods are detrimental to your health and increase the risk of disease. Avoid processed foods, especially foods with added sugar, refined carbohydrates, or vegetable oils such as corn or canola oil.

- **Reduce carbohydrates.** You need an appropriate amount of protein, carbs, and fat in your diet (the three primary macronutrients). The optimal amount of each depends on your activity levels and dietary goals. However, most people in the developed world eat too many carbs compared with protein and fat.

- **Get plenty of micronutrients.** You gain micronutrients by eating a balanced diet of nutritious whole foods from animals and plants.

- **Measure your food intake.** Weigh and measure your foods and log your intake, at least for a limited period of time. You will gain greater awareness of the amount and composition of the foods you eat. This will lead to you improving your dietary habits.

- **Experiment.** There is no one-size-fits-all. Genetics and gut bacteria differ among people and regions. This makes certain foods healthy for some but problematic for others. You will need to figure out the best diet for yourself by gauging how your body responds to different foods.

Practical eating strategies

These principles still leave many questions unanswered. What should be the proportions of the macronutrients? How much should I eat? How often should I eat? Which foods should I get my proteins, carbs, and fats from? And should I weigh and measure my foods, or count calories?

Most CrossFit athletes fill in these blanks by adhering to the Paleo Diet or the Zone Diet, or some mixture of the two. Both provide a more detailed implementation of the general dietary principles outlined in this section.

There are countless free websites with good and detailed information on both of these diets. There, you can find meal suggestions and more detailed info on the philosophy behind each. To get you started, I will provide an overview of the key elements of both diets.

The Paleo Diet

The Paleo Diet is based on the idea that over the course of human history, our bodies have adapted to eating foods from our natural environment. Conversely, our bodies are not adapted to man-made foods from the agricultural and industrial revolutions. This means that some foods, grains in particular, are poorly tolerated by our intestines and are detrimental to our health.

On the Paleo Diet, you eat only whole, unprocessed foods. Additionally, the goal is to exclude foods that irritate the gut and cause excessive inflammation or blood sugar spikes. Since gaining popularity around 30 years ago, the Paleo Diet has evolved along with new insights in nutrition science. There are now a few variants of this diet, but three types of foods are almost always excluded:

- **Grains** (e.g., wheat, rye, barley, rice, corn). Skipping grains is the most important component of the Paleo Diet. The reasoning is that modern grains have little to do with whole foods. They consist of carbohydrates devoid of nutrients, which causes metabolic problems and disease. Additionally, they contain antinutrients and inflammatory proteins such as gluten. These can irritate and inflame the gut, contributing to digestive problems and autoimmune disorders.

- **Beans and legumes** (e.g., soybeans, peanuts, peas, lentils). These foods are high in phytic acid, which prevents absorption of the foods' nutrients. They also contain lectins, which can cause gut problems for some people. Soybeans and peanuts are particularly unhealthy because of other toxins as well, so Paleo adherents strictly avoid these.

- **Seed oils** (e.g., soybean oil, canola oil). These processed oils are used by almost all restaurants and as cooking oils in most homes. They are oxidized, which makes them highly inflammatory. They are also high in omega-6, which, in excess, causes a wide range of inflammatory problems.

Additionally, on the Paleo Diet, the following foods are either fully skipped or reduced in consumption by some of those who follow it:

- **Dairy.** Some Paleo eaters skip dairy completely. Lactose is poorly tolerated by many, and dairy foods have an insulin-promoting effect that can contribute to metabolic problems. Those who include dairy only do so partially. They stick to full-fat, fermented products like yogurt and cheese, as well as butter. Dairy-based protein powders are also consumed by many athletes; these will be covered in the Supplements chapter.

- **Nuts and seeds.** Like legumes, nuts and seeds contain phytic acid, making it preferable to soak them in water overnight before eating to break down the acid. For most people, this is a bigger hassle than simply skipping these foods. Additionally, nuts and seeds are high in polyunsaturated and omega-6 fats, both of which should be minimized in modern diets. There are two exceptions to this: macadamia nuts and chestnuts, both of which are safe to eat, as they are low in both phytic acid and omega-6.

- **Alcohol.** Beer is skipped altogether because it is grain-based and contains unwanted residues, such as gluten. However, wine and spirits are consumed sporadically or in moderation by some.

After reading this, you may be wondering if there is anything that you can actually eat. In fact, it is important to focus more on what you can eat instead of the foods you are skipping. Without this mindset, you will start to feel like you are denying yourself these foods. This undermines your commitment and makes you revert to your previous habits. Here are the foods you can eat freely on the Paleo Diet:

- **Unprocessed meats:** includes both lean and fatty cuts of most animals; grass-fed animals are preferred
- **Fish** and other seafood
- **Fruits**
- **Vegetables**
- **Eggs**
- **Herbs and spices**
- **Coffee and tea**
- **Various fats**: olive oil, coconut oil, animal fat, and avocados

Used creatively, these foods will provide you with more than enough variety for a lifetime of healthy eating. Additionally, the diet actually gives you more freedom than a regular diet in other aspects. According to the Paleo philosophy, before the agricultural revolution, the human body automatically regulated appetite, weight, and hunger. This means that if you stick to the foods allowed above, you are free to eat as much as you want, whenever you want, and can still expect to improve your health, performance, and physique.

The Zone Diet

The Paleo and Zone Diets share many common traits. However, they have one key difference. Paleo mostly focuses on quality by prescribing which foods to eat, but not their portioning and timing. Zone, however, emphasizes quantity through the measuring of portions and timing of meals.

Having eaten countless meals over our lives, we are creatures of strong habits when it comes to food. The simple act of measuring and recording what we eat increases our awareness of what and how much we actually eat over the course of the day.

This is the central premise of the Zone Diet. By weighing and measuring our food intake, we can balance our intake of the three different macronutrients. This, in turn, reduces excessive inflammation and stabilizes our hormones, leading to both increased overall health and higher performance in the box.

Measuring every meal is a big commitment. However, the effect on your fitness level can be profound. If the commitment still seems too high, start by weighing and measuring your foods for a week. Just that will give you a better feel for the amount of macronutrients included in your meals.

As mentioned, CrossFitters who focus on nutrition often adhere to a mixture of the Paleo and Zone Diets. They measure and weigh their foods, at least for a few weeks, and stick to Paleo foods as the ingredients for their meals. If you want to improve in CrossFit but still haven't tried improving your dietary habits, doing so might be one of your biggest opportunities.

Chapter 9: Lifestyle

The second component to consider for effective recovery is your lifestyle. Are you getting enough sleep? How are your stress levels? Do you drink too much? Are you sedentary or do you move during your day? These are all parts of your lifestyle that affect your athletic performance. We will discuss each one in this chapter.

Sleep

Adequate sleep is an integral part of any effective training regimen. High training loads call for more sleep than otherwise. Without enough sleep, your recovery will be slower and less pronounced. Furthermore, a lack of sleep will impair you mentally, reducing motivation, focus, and intensity in your training sessions.

Lack of sleep is holding many people back. According to the Centers for Disease Control and Prevention, a third of Americans sleep less than seven hours per day. This is attributed to modern culture, most notably stress, stimulants, and electronics. These things disrupt our body's natural sleep mechanism and cause us to miss out on our body's cue to go to bed when we need to.

Luckily, there are solutions to this problem. Here are a few things you can do to improve your sleep patterns:

- **Go to bed and wake up at the same time every day.** This includes the weekends.

- **Make your bedroom sleep-friendly.** Remove all sources of light and noise, adjust room temperature to around 65–68°F (18–20°C), and ensure good air circulation.

- **Avoid electronics at night.** Do not look at electronic screens when bedtime is approaching. This includes TVs, computers, smartphones, and tablets. The blue light from electronic screens interferes with your body's production of melatonin, a sleep-promoting hormone.

- **Avoid stimulants and large meals before bedtime.** This includes alcohol, caffeine, and nicotine. Note that chocolate often includes a significant amount of caffeine.

Hydration

The importance of hydration for athletic performance has been realized increasingly in the last few years. Lack of proper hydration can decrease the viscosity between layers of skin, fascia, muscles, and ligaments. This reduces mobility and increases inertia when we move.

Your body gives you a good estimate of your hydration levels through the color of your urine. A clear or very light yellow color indicates that you are well hydrated. But if the color is a darker yellow or orange, you need to drink more fluids.

Another method you can use to determine how much you need to drink is to weigh yourself before and after a workout. The difference will indicate how much water you need to replenish.

To increase hydration, you can add electrolytes to your fluids. A common method is to add a pinch of salt or lemon/lime juice to your water. This is more hydrating than drinking only water by itself.

Additionally, make sure you don't go into a workout thirsty. Drinking a glass or two of water 30–60 minutes before a workout should ensure you remain hydrated throughout the workout.

Alcohol

As you already know, alcohol can have a negative effect on athletic performance. This is especially true with an intense fitness program such as CrossFit. Alcohol disrupts your sleep patterns and alters your hormone levels, inhibiting recovery. It also has a dehydrating effect, with the negative consequences already described. Finally, alcohol consists of "empty calories" devoid of micronutrients, so it has a negative effect on your diet. In summary, you should probably skip it completely if you are serious about your training.

However, with the prevalence of alcohol in modern culture, it is possible that you will keep drinking despite these effects. In that case, consider this research. An interesting study tested the effect of different levels of alcohol consumption on athletes.[1] It concluded that alcohol consumption of 1 gram per kilogram of body weight had a significant negative effect on muscle recovery and growth. However, 0.5 grams per kg had very little effect.

Let's put the results of this study in understandable terms. One alcoholic drink, such as a bottle of beer or a glass of wine, contains approximately 14 grams of alcohol. So the lower amount of 0.5 grams per kg corresponds to two drinks for a lightweight female (125 lbs. or 57 kg), or three drinks for a medium-build male (185 lbs. or 84 kg).

---

1 M. J. Barnes, "Alcohol: Impact on Sports Performance and Recovery in Male Athletes," Sports Medicine 44, no. 7 (2014): 909, doi: 10.1007/s40279-014-0192-8.

This study illustrates how the negative effect of alcohol grows disproportionately as you drink more. If you choose to drink, do your best to stay at or below these amounts to ensure you don't undo your progress.

Movement

No matter how active you are in CrossFit, most of your waking hours are spent outside of the box. To illustrate, let's assume you sleep for 8 hours every night and train for 1.5 hours five times per week. This would mean that training would constitute 7 percent of your waking hours. So, even if you are very active, 93 percent of your time will be spent on other activities.

Increasingly, these other activities have come to mean sitting still in a chair or a couch. A recent study using smartphone data estimates that just 3 percent of our waking hours are spent exercising, while 39 percent is spent on light-intensity activity and the remaining 58 percent is spent sedentary.[2] The conclusion is that the average person spends the majority of waking hours sitting still.

Exercise doesn't undo the negative effects of prolonged sitting. A recent study refers to those who regularly work out but are primarily sedentary as *Active Couch*

2 Neville Owen, et al., "Sedentary Behavior: Emerging Evidence for a New Health Risk," Mayo Clinic Proceedings 85 (December 2010): 1138–41, doi: http://dx.doi.org/10.4065/mcp.2010.0444.

Potatoes. It concluded that despite regular exercise, prolonged sitting hours still had a detrimental effect on their metabolism, including higher blood pressure and blood sugar levels.[3] So, the harmful effects of sedentary behavior cannot be undone with training.

You can make simple changes to reduce prolonged sitting. For example, try standing at your workstation in the office, walking or biking instead of driving shorter distances, or standing up regularly to stretch or move around when sitting at home. A few simple changes like this can go a long way.

Nature

The last lifestyle adjustment to consider is to spend more time outdoors. In recent years, studies have highlighted the benefits of spending time outside for both mental and physical health. Among the effects are decreased stress, improved concentration, boosted immunity, increased energy levels, and improved sleep.[4] These effects occurred despite the studies'

3 Owen, et al., "Too Much Sitting: The Population-Health Science of Sedentary Behavior," Exercise and Sports Sciences Reviews 38, no. 3 (July 2010): 105–13, doi: 10.1097/JES.0b013e3181e373a2.
4 Beata Mostafavi, "Walking Off Depression and Beating Stress Outdoors? Nature Group Walks Linked to Improved Mental Health" (press release), University of Michigan, September 23, 2014,
http://www.uofmhealth.org/news/archive/ 201409/walking-depression-and-beating-stress-outdoors-nature-group; "Immerse Yourself in a Forest for Better Health," New York State Department of Environmental

control groups moving or exercising indoors for comparison. Thus, being in the outdoors is beneficial in itself.

Experiment with simple activities such as walks or light jogs on your rest days, running interval workouts, or training outside when you can. See whether these changes help you reach your training goals faster.

Conservation, http://www.dec.ny.gov/lands/90720.html; Frances Kuo and Andrea Faber Taylor, "A Potential Natural Treatment for Attention-Deficit/Hyperactivity Disorder: Evidence from a National Study," *American Journal of Public Health* 94, no. 9 (September 2004): 1580-6, https://www.ncbi.nlm.nih.gov/pmc/articles/PMC1448497.

Chapter 10: Supplements

The final topic we will cover regarding recovery is dietary supplements. But before we get into the details, always remember that improving your diet and lifestyle will result in greater improvements than adding supplements on top of inadequate habits in those domains. So, most likely, following the advice in the previous chapters is more important for you than anything that follows here.

We need to keep this fact constantly in mind. Various companies continuously market all sorts of supplements that are promised to help us. This is evident on the social media accounts of CrossFit athletes, many of whom promote supplements and their beneficial effects (usually with a discount code included) more than the importance of a healthy diet.

Without awareness of this bias in our information supply, those who want to improve may focus too much on supplements while neglecting more important factors, such as nutrition and lifestyle. If your main goal is to improve your long-term health, consider skipping most or all supplements and seeking to get everything you need from your diet.

Nevertheless, some supplements can certainly help you reach your goals more quickly. But not all of them are created equal. I recommend that you always do two things before purchasing a supplement you are considering.

First, read up on what the research says and decide for yourself whether you think it justifies the purchase. There are good websites to do this, such as Examine.com, whose team has read through hundreds of research papers and summarized the results in plain English.

Second, but no less important, review the quality of the particular brand you are considering. There are countless brands selling poor quality or even fraudulent supplements that don't contain at all what they claim. Labdoor.com is the biggest company specializing in testing supplements from specific brands and would be a good place to start.

But enough with the disclaimers—let's discuss the supplements themselves. There are five supplements you should consider: creatine, caffeine, protein, omega-3, and certain vitamins and minerals. Evidence for other supplements is mixed or limited, but a discussion on them is also included in case you want to dig deeper.

Supplements to consider

Creatine

Creatine should be at the top of your supplement list. It plays a vital role in the generation of energy in muscles through the anaerobic system. Creatine is naturally produced by the body and also obtained from food, primarily stored in muscles.

Supplementing creatine has been popular since the '90s, and, unlike most supplements, which quickly fade in popularity, it is still going strong. The reason is simply that the supplement works. Scientific studies have repeatedly confirmed its positive effects on training and performance.

The benefits of creatine apply particularly to CrossFit. Creatine has been demonstrated in numerous studies to increase both strength and weightlifting performance. A comprehensive metastudy that reviewed the result of 22 scientific studies found that strength increased by 8 percent on average and weightlifting performance by 14 percent.[1]

Creatine is a safe supplement without significant side effects, even after long-term use. Only those with kidney disease, high blood pressure, or liver disease should avoid it as a supplement. Additionally, avoid taking creatine with NSAIDs (nonsteroidal anti-inflammatory drugs) such as ibuprofen or naproxen, as together it can increase stress on your kidneys.

Caffeine

This supplement needs little introduction as you most likely are already consuming it daily. In addition to coffee and tea, pre-workout drinks containing caffeine are also popular.

Caffeine, like creatine, has been widely studied and its effects demonstrated. In the context of training, its effects are mainly increased focus and effort. In one study, caffeine helped athletes lift slightly greater weights.[2] The reason is the stimulating effect of caffeine,

1 E. S. Rawson and J. S. Volek, "Effects of Creatine Supplementation and Resistance Training on Muscle Strength and Weightlifting Performance" (review), *Journal of Strength and Conditioning Research* 17, no. 4 (November 2003): 822–31, PubMed PMID: 14636102.
2 M. J. Duncan, M. Smith, K. Cook, and R. S. James, "The Acute Effect of a Caffeine-Containing Energy Drink on Mood State, Readiness to Invest Effort, and Resistance Exercise to Failure," *Journal of Strength and Conditioning Research* 26, no. 10 (October 2012): 2858–65, doi: 10.1519/JSC.0b013e318241e124.

which causes you to be more focused and "pumped up" for a few hours after consumption.

The downside of caffeine is that we build up tolerance to it, so frequent consumption negates this boosting effect. This means that if you regularly drink coffee or caffeinated tea throughout the day, more caffeine before a training session will have little or no effect. For caffeine to work as a training supplement, you should limit its consumption to before a workout.

Protein powder

Protein powder is technically processed food, not a supplement. It is one of the three macronutrients but in powdered form. You should supplement with protein powder only if you are fine with deviating from the Paleo principle of eating only whole foods. Most protein powders are made from milk, so when you have a protein drink, you are usually drinking a dairy product. Protein is commonly supplemented by athletes, often combined with creatine.

The three most common types of protein are whey, casein, and soy. Whey and casein are dairy based, with whey being the most popular. Whey is synthesized quickly and thus commonly consumed immediately after a workout. The scientific evidence on the effects of whey is somewhat mixed, with some studies showing a benefit for muscle growth and recovery but others showing little effect.[3]

In scientific studies of protein powders, the problem is often the difficulty of performing double-blind studies. If a researcher has two groups, with one group consuming protein powder after a workout and the other consuming nothing, the former will most likely show better results. But this does not prove that protein powders are effective. Consuming a glass of milk post-workout could very well provide you with the same benefits of protein powders, as it contains both whey and casein proteins in addition to other macronutrients.

Thus, protein powder is not superior to whole foods when it comes to obtaining your macronutrients. The primary benefit is convenience for those who are short on time or dedication. If you feel like you would benefit from a convenient source of protein to meet your daily goals, powdered proteins are an affordable and convenient way to do that.

Omega-3

In the average modern diet, a person consumes much more of omega-6 fatty acids than omega-3 fatty acids.

---

3 S. M. Pasiakos, H. R. Lieberman, and T. M. McLellan, "Effects of Protein Supplements on Muscle Damage, Soreness, and Recovery of Muscle Function and Physical Performance: A Systematic Review," *Sports Medicine* 44, no. 5 (May 2014): 655, doi: 10.1007/s40279-013-0137-7.

But before the agricultural revolution, the ratio between these two was very similar. This change has led to an imbalance that can contribute to increased levels of inflammation.

The idea behind supplementing with omega-3 is to restore this balance. There is some scientific evidence that points to omega-3 supplementation reducing both triglyceride levels in the blood and inflammation throughout the body, making it a popular supplement in recent years.

You could obtain more omega-3 by eating fatty fish at least two times per week. But, like with protein powders, many resort to supplementing for practical reasons.

Omega-3 is often obtained by consuming fish oil. Recently, krill oil has become popular as well. Some studies suggest that the fatty acids from krill oil are better absorbed by the body than those from fish oil. Additionally, krill is lower in the food chain than fish, which leads to lower concentrations of toxins.

A growing number of studies show that omega-3 supplementation has benefits while the side effects are limited. So, if you don't eat a lot of fatty fish, chances are your health would benefit from supplementing with omega-3.

Vitamins and minerals

Many individuals are low in certain vitamins and/or minerals. The most common deficiencies are vitamin D, vitamin B12, zinc, and magnesium. If you are serious about improving your performance, consider ordering blood work to check your vitamin and mineral levels and identify specific deficiencies. I did this a few times, and the tests revealed that my D and B12 vitamin levels were too low. After supplementing in response, I have felt my energy levels increase, both inside the box and also in daily life.

What you should not do is take multivitamins. If you follow a reasonably healthy diet, you probably already receive most vitamins and minerals you need from food, and the effectiveness of multivitamins has not been demonstrated. So stick to a targeted approach and only supplement with what you actually need.

Supplements you probably don't need

The supplement industry constantly develops new products. Over the last few decades, countless new supplements have become popular for a short time. Most of them fade into oblivion once the scientific literature and athletes' experience together conclude that they provide no benefit. But creatine was one exception, popularized in the 1990s by a supplements company and withstanding the test of time ever since.

So some of these new compounds may provide real benefits. We just don't know enough about them yet to be sure.

There are a few supplements in the CrossFit universe that fall into this category. The following are the most common:

- **HMB:** This is a naturally produced compound that has been demonstrated to increase muscle size and strength as well as enhance recovery from a workout. The compound does this primarily by inhibiting the breakdown of proteins in muscles. It is used medically to prevent muscle loss in older adults and is becoming increasingly popular with athletes. Studies have not found any significant side effects, even from long-term use. However, the compound is metabolized from leucine, a branched-chain amino acid (BCAA), which appears to be more effective in promoting muscle growth than HMB.

- **BCAAs:** Branched-chain amino acids have been demonstrated to be beneficial for muscle growth and repair. But some studies have shown that supplementing with whey protein, which contains all the essential amino acids, including the BCAAs, is as effective or even more so.

- **Glutamine:** A naturally occurring amino acid, glutamine mostly seems to aid performance in athletes deficient in it due to either low protein intake or very high workloads. Additionally, it is already included in whey protein.

- **Beta-alanine:** This is a version of alanine, which is an amino acid. Is has been shown to increase muscular endurance, but the effect is small and the research is not extensive. Additionally, the compound is prevalent in animal foods, so another way to increase it would be to eat meat or dairy.

- **Melatonin:** Taking melatonin is a safe, nonaddictive way to promote sleep. However, the body regulates melatonin production on its own, so supplementation should only be considered when traveling or working night or evening shifts.

- **Nitric Oxide:** This compound can increase muscular endurance and strength. It is popular to include nitric oxide in pre-workout drinks. However, the precursor to nitric oxide is arginine, which is already included in whey protein and can also be obtained from foods such as nuts, fruit, meat, and dairy.

Many will disagree with the preceding list. After reviewing both the literature and the debate on all these supplements, one thing is clear: there is little consensus on most of these products. Views range all the way from considering all supplements as unhealthy because they are not real foods, to recommending most or all of the supplements I've mentioned, plus others not included on this list.

So do not think of the text here as an authoritative source on what to supplement with. For you to make an informed decision, you need to read the opposing views and decide on your own.

Conclusion

One of my favorite parts about CrossFit is the complexity. The aim of the sport has many aspects, each of which requires different considerations in training. As a consequence, improvement is not only about training hard but equally so about training smart. Equipped with the knowledge from this book, you are now in possession of a toolbox you can use to do exactly that.

Enjoy your training, and best of luck in the next Open.

Glossary of Terms

Following are some of the key terms used specifically in CrossFit. Descriptions of specific movements are not included. If you want to learn about a particular movement mentioned in the book, free online videos on CrossFit.com or YouTube are a superior resource to a text description.

Affiliate: A gym that is licensed by CrossFit Inc. as a legitimate facility for CrossFit training.

AMRAP: Acronym for "as many reps/rounds as possible." This is one type of workout in which the athlete finishes as much work as possible within a specified amount of time.

Box: A CrossFit affiliate gym. The name refers to the barebones nature of many affiliates, because all that is needed is floor space and some free weights.

CrossFit Games: An annual competition, held by CrossFit Inc., that anyone can participate in. The competition is divided into three stages: the Open, the Regionals, and the Games. In the final stage, athletes from all over the world compete for the title of "Fittest on Earth."

CrossFit Open: The first stage of the CrossFit Games. Here, athletes compete online by submitting scores from workouts performed at affiliates or recorded on video. Anyone can participate, and 500,000 people did so in 2018.

CrossFit Regionals: The second stage of the CrossFit Games, where only the top athletes from the Open can participate. The Regionals are held in a number of different locations all over the world. The top athletes from each region advance to the Games.

Globo gym: A traditional non–CrossFit gym, where barbells cannot be dropped, treadmills and machines dominate the floor space, and mirrors are common.

Leaderboard: An online Whiteboard for the CrossFit Open. The Leaderboard is published on CrossFit.com and ranks every Open athlete based on workout performance. See also Whiteboard.

Metcon: Shorthand for "metabolic conditioning." This is any type of workout in which an athlete performs work as fast as possible. This develops both the aerobic and anaerobic systems that metabolize energy. Metcons are often included in the WOD, but not always. Sometimes, WODs only include skill- or strength-based components.

RX: The most challenging version of a workout. The symbol is the same as is used for medical drug prescriptions, highlighting CrossFit's philosophy of improving health with a daily dose of training. See also Scaled.

Scaled: CrossFit is designed to work for all athletes, regardless of their level of fitness or ability. Accordingly, workouts usually come in more manageable Scaled versions in addition to the more challenging RX versions. Additionally, athletes are encouraged to "scale" all workouts to their level of ability, for example, by using lower weights or doing simpler movements. See also RX.

Whiteboard: The Whiteboard is where members of a CrossFit affiliate write their results for the WOD. This can be an actual whiteboard on the facilities or an electronic whiteboard through a website or an app. The idea behind the Whiteboard is to provide athletes with measurability of their results. See also Leaderboard.

WOD: Acronym for "Workout of the Day." This is the basis of CrossFit programming. Affiliate boxes host WOD classes daily, and CrossFit.com also publishes a WOD online.

Manufactured by Amazon.ca
Bolton, ON

10542621R00090